HEALTHFUL
COMMUNICATIONS

Healthful Communications, Inc.
Juno Beach Professional Building
13700 U.S. Highway One, Suite #202A
Juno Beach, FL 33408
(561) 626-3293
www.healthfulcommunications.com

Publisher
Brian M. Connolly

Associate Publisher
Eric Zayes

Managing Editor
Lynn Komlenic

Contributing Editors
Stephen R.M. Jones
Catharine Rambeau

Director of Research
Scott Treadway, Ph.D.

Typography
Yanileysi Bailes

Cover Art and Design
Jim Scattaregia

coolingtheplanet.org

This publication is printed on Recycled Paper and with soy-based inks. Alternative First, Inc. replenishes more than the amount of trees required to print this publication, through www.coolingtheplanet.org.

www.papaschoice.com

GENERATION A.D.D.

NATURAL SOLUTIONS
FOR BREAKING THE
PRESCRIPTION ADDICTION

DR. MICHAEL PAPA

Dedication

This book is dedicated to all the parents who are willing to do whatever needs to be done to raise healthy children and families. We honor those of you with the courage to ask the questions and question the answers for the future of generations to come. You are the shepherds of healthy families, guiding them along the correct and natural path, rather than following the highway of mediocrity without question or pause. In a society that is dependent on drugs and blindly follows the newest chemical trends, thank you for being good shepherds in a healthy and more vibrant way of living. This book is also dedicated to my lovely and supportive wife, Adrienne, and our children Bianca, Isabella and Beckett. It is because of all of you that I am inspired to do all I can to create healthy families everywhere.

Table of Contents

INTRODUCTION

Over nearly two decades of counseling parents of children with Attention Deficit Disorder and Attention Deficit Hyperactivity Disorder (ADD/ADHD), and treating both children and parents, I have found that many parents worry deeply about putting their children on drug programs. I fully share this concern. I believe it is vital to look carefully and cautiously at all sides of any issue involving our children's health, and particularly when it comes to a diagnosis or treatment of ADD or ADHD.

Working with parents and children over the past 18 years, I have found answers to their problems. The key is to ask the right questions – and listen to the answers! Drugs are *not* your only solution and *should not be your first choice* in cases of ADD or ADHD. Why? In a nutshell, drugs often create worse problems than the ones they are supposed to solve, and sometimes their use is outright dangerous.

First, let's take the time for the important step of looking at daily habits, routines and other factors that can be a root cause of symptoms. These can include:

- Poor nutrition
- Mineral, vitamin, and nutrient deficiencies
- High blood sugar levels

- High consumption of caffeine, sugar or other stimulating products
- Poor sleep habits
- Insufficient exercise
- Food allergies
- Environmental hazards – including toxins that may be present in your living room, basement, kitchen, lawn or schoolroom
- Too much time spent in front of the television or computer, and playing video games
- An emotionally stressful living environment or situation

All of the above points, along with other considerations that I will address in later chapters, should be examined and fully exhausted ***before any medications are given***. You can also go to my website www.papaschoice.com for a more in-depth discussion on symptoms and first steps.

The first natural choice is to adjust lifestyle and nutritional factors before considering a jump into dangerous medications. If you do not address proper nutrition and lifestyle choices then signs of ADD/ADHD will most likely continue to appear and no magic drug can prevent them!

Of course, it is much easier to give your child the drug your physician prescribes than to face the challenge of making the necessary dietary and lifestyle changes, but then what? You might be lucky and see some results from the medication, but these are likely to last only a short time. Where does this leave you? *Right back with the same problem.*

If you are really serious about eliminating ADD/ADHD in your children, you must not only consider breaking out of your comfort zones regarding nutrition and lifestyle, you must also make the time to educate yourself on the best choices for your children and your family.

Yes, this involves effort – but the effort will be well worthwhile. There is no greater satisfaction or reward than giving your child the gift of health. The natural approach I recommend will not create unpleasant side effects, nor carry the risk of addiction and other dangers associated with drug therapies. Drugs used to control ADD/ADHD are dangerous and can create a lifetime of illness and dependency. Your children's lives – and your own – are precious. Always seek alternatives to drugs. Talk to your physician or health care provider and make sure you exhaust every alternative before stepping onto the slippery slope of a drug medication program which you may never get off.

In this book I will show you healthy and intelligent alternatives to control and eliminate the symptoms associated with ADD/ADHD *naturally*. We will discuss the causes of ADD/ADHD, their signs and symptoms, and natural approaches to treatment and prevention including a balanced lifestyle and proper nutrition – which I consider to be at least 50 percent, and sometimes much more, of the battle to eliminate ADD/ADHD symptoms. I will also discuss the dangers of medication and review the drugs that are commonly prescribed for ADD/ADHD.

1
The Doping Epidemic

As I sat in the hospital anxiously waiting for my wife to give birth to our third child, my mind was full of thoughts about the miracle of childbirth, and also of my responsibility to protect and shelter this newborn life as he develops, providing the best parental care and guidance, including health care, that I possibly could.

I have been in practice for over 17 years and now, with three children of my own, I feel an additional public responsibility: to share my experience as a doctor with other parents who, like me, want to raise healthier and well-developed children.

Over the years I have encountered many parents who are concerned about their young child or teenager who seems to lack concentration, or feels fatigued, or is overweight. I am often asked what ADD and ADHD really are. Parents will say "They sent my child home from school because of his behavior," or "The school wants my child to see a psychologist," or "They want me to medicate my child." They ask "What are my options?" or "Please help me with my child's symptoms!"

For the sake of my patients and my own family I began researching and developing options and natural alternatives for my patients concerned about ADD/ADHD. Over the last 10 years I have developed a successful plan to help them reduce symptoms, and in some cases eliminate them entirely, and help address the concerns they have.

It is estimated that 6 million children in the United States are currently prescribed Ritalin or another drug to control the symptoms of ADD/ADHD.

I have had many opportunities to listen to a large number of children who have been put on psychotropic medications and each year I seemed to be talking to many more of these children.

In the United States, medicating our children has become by far the most popular way of dealing with these conditions. If we can talk of an epidemic of ADD/ADHD, we can also talk of a drugging epidemic. Psychotropic prescription drugs are given as freely as candy to vast numbers of children, and doctors are writing these prescriptions routinely and expeditiously, without a thorough examination of the child's individual case and circumstances.

Through my clinical work, I came to see that these drugs simply mask the symptoms of ADD/ADHD rather than address the core causes of the conditions. The medication solution, issued by medical personnel and blindly accepted or supported by frightened and uneducated parents, is actually hiding the *real* problem rather than fixing it. It became very clear to me that the public is being misled by the medical community and profiteering multi-national pharmaceutical companies and brainwashed into believing that drugs could solve the problems of ADD/ADHD. Worst of all, the children have no choice. They are victims of our society's ignorant and erroneous belief in "better medicine through chemistry." Needless to say, I became very angry about the whole situation. It was at this point that I resolved to attempt to reverse the prevailing tide and to end the mistreatment of those suffering from ADHD.

JUST SAY NO!

Not many years ago our national government started a campaign to encourage young people to "Just say no to drugs." This was a wonderful initiative, meant to protect our children from the very real dangers of street drugs. Now, it would seem, there is an unofficial national strategy that is exactly the reverse, one that encourages children and adults to "say yes" to drugs to alleviate *any* illness or disease, not just ADD/ADHD. In fact, the long lines at school nurses' stations would indicate that we are indeed in the throes of an epidemic. These drugs, like street drugs, carry very real dangers, including lifelong dependence. And while they are legal substances, they too are undermining the health, welfare and stability of those who use them. The strategy of using drugs as primary care is being inflicted on children in the name of behavioral control. It might appear to be a simple solution, but it actually represents a risky shift in our attitude toward legal drugs.

Interestingly, the sting of this reality has been softened by terminology: Medical and marketing professionals now prefer the much more passive label of "meds." We naturally assume that that prescription drugs are safer and less addictive than street drugs, but in fact they can be equally dangerous and addictive, and even more so. In my opinion, any change in our attitude toward drugs should be viewed with great caution, especially where our children are concerned. Children are vulnerable – in particular because of their underdeveloped immune systems – and highly dependent. I agree that we should "Just say no to drugs" – including medication to control our own or our children's behavior!

We have been too quick to embrace "chemical parenting," following the lead of the big pharmaceutical companies who want us to believe that drugs are the only viable first choice to helping children with ADD/ADHD. This may be good for supporting the multibillion-dollar business models of big drug companies, but it is bad for our children.

I do believe that drugs can be helpful where there are real requirements for them, especially short-term emergency necessities when no alternatives are available. But a natural approach, beginning at home, should always be the first choice. Drugs are a very serious and potentially dangerous choice that should always come *second*, only after every natural alternative has been exhausted.

ADD/ADHD was first described many years ago, but only in recent decades has it been recognized as a widespread problem. Have we suddenly developed a nation of kids with new mental disorders?

I believe not. The current prevalence of ADD/ADHD is the result of a long process of societal corruption, including bad foods, bad influences, bad entertainment, and many other factors. Parents today are under more stress and time constraints than in the past and, as a result, now find it incredibly difficult to deal with the relational and cultural problems of their children. Instead, they turn to drugs like Ritalin – a chemical crutch – because they seem to provide an easy solution.

The problem with this approach is that it means giving up our real parenting responsibilities in favor of drugs that are nothing more than a "chemical babysitter" – and a sorely inadequate one at that. Using chemicals creates more problems for children in

According to the Congressional Testimony of Terrance Woodworth, a deputy director of the Drug Enforcement Administration, the number of prescriptions written for methylphenidate [Ritalin] has increased by a factor of five since 1991. About 80 percent of the 11 million prescriptions doctors write for that medication each year treat childhood ADHD, he said. In addition, production of Adderall and Dexedrine, also used to treat ADHD, has risen 2,000 percent in nine years.

www.education-world.com/a_issues/issues148a.shtml

the long run: Physically, their immune systems are weakened, which increases their susceptibility to illness. They may also experience negative side-effects and develop a dependency on drugs. Mentally and emotionally, they are vulnerable to "chemical dependency" attitudes that result in an undeveloped and immature coping mechanism into adulthood. When children are "doped up," they do not develop a healthy ability to respond and relate to the world at large. The resulting feelings of helplessness, anxiety and depression, as they grow older, ironically perpetuate and may even increase the need for this "pain-killing" substance – and so the addiction continues. This spiral can lead to significant problems in later life, including problems with work and relationships.

Various societal factors have contributed to the problem of doping our children. For example, economic realities force both parents to work longer hours and spend less quality time with their children. Schoolteachers are under pressure with larger classrooms and more children to supervise – and they sometimes ask parents to consider putting kids on drugs simply to create a classroom with easier-to-control children!

Aside from medications supplied by parents through doctors, children themselves are taking more illegal drugs voluntarily to combat the lack of parental supervision. A Columbia University study shows that isolation from parents and schedules that keep kids from constructive "quality time" with mom and dad are key contributing factors in the use of drugs and alcohol among middle-class children. "Suniya S. Luthar, a professor of Psychology and Education at Columbia's Teacher's College, first studied an older group of suburban high school students as a control group to compare with inner-city youth," explains UPI reporter Lou Marano. "The suburban 10th-graders had significantly higher levels of every kind of substance use – cigarettes, alcohol, marijuana and hard drugs – than did their inner-city counterparts."

Puzzled by the results, researchers went back into the field. They turned up very similar results for junior-high kids as well. It emerged that parents, too busy with work and outside events, are not spending enough time parenting and so the kids abuse drugs.

Parents who cannot spend time with their children often resort to doping their troubled kids with legal prescription drugs obtained from their family physician. This never works out well and the children suffer. It would be better to consider lifestyle changes and safer alternative-health approaches – even where it is not possible for parents to spend more time with their children.

We all want our children to be healthy and we do not want to contribute to a generation of drug-dependent kids who may become drug-dependent adults. Yes, drugs can be very useful at times, when used according to carefully considered physician's recommendations, or when carefully prescribed plans and emergency approaches are necessary, but let's not get confused. The interests of large, multi-national, profit-hungry drug companies do not always coincide with the best interests of our precious families.

2
What Is ADD/ADHD?

To begin, let's review some of the common definitions and symptoms that I use to determine the presence and treatment of ADD/ADHD conditions in children and adults.

Attention Deficit Disorder (ADD) and Attention Deficit Hyperactivity Disorder (ADHD) have become pervasive in North America. They can appear as a mild condition or as a severe disability. ADD/ADHD was determined by a vote of American Psychiatric Association (APA) psychiatrists to be a mental illness, and in 1987 was added to the Diagnostic and Statistical Manual of Mental Disorders (a reference manual published by the APA covering all known mental health disorders of children and adults).

In the United States, ADD/ADHD affects five percent or more of all school children and an even larger percentage of adults. As a result, the overall health of children and adults in our country is at stake. The personal, societal, and economic costs of a child or adult's mental dysfunction are incalculable. It is safe to say that every member of society is affected directly or indirectly by ADD/ADHD and that everyone concerned should take action now to protect our children's mental health, our mental health and our future.

ADD, Attention Deficit Disorder, is associated with the inability to focus attention on a task, project or other activity. It is a condition related to difficulty sitting still, paying attention or controlling impulsive behavior. In some cases, these symptoms are persistent and interfere with daily life, including activities at home, school, social engagements, and work settings.

ADHD, Attention Deficit Hyperactivity Disorder, is usually expressed as inappropriate activities and impulsive behaviors such as hyperactivity. ADHD is classed as a neurobiological disorder affecting many schoolchildren. But it is important to remember that if symptoms of ADHD are left untreated they may continue into adulthood.

Some signs of ADD and/or ADHD are:

- Squirming in one's seat, fidgety behavior with hands and feet
- Difficulty remaining seated
- Not keeping hands to oneself
- Difficulty waiting one's turn (in games or group activities)
- Blurting out answers out of turn or before a question is completed
- Difficulty following instructions
- Difficulty sustaining attention in tasks or activities
- Shifting from one uncompleted task to another
- Difficulty playing quietly
- Excessive talking
- Interrupting or intruding on others
- Not listening to what is being said
- Forgetting things necessary for tasks or activities
- Engaging in physically dangerous activities without considering consequences

THE DIAGNOSIS

Almost every child will exhibit some of the behaviors listed above at times; this does not mean that they have ADD/ADHD. A diagnosis of ADD/ADHD should be determined by a trusted and trained health professional with experience in recognizing and treating ADD/ADHD conditions. Children who are diagnosed with ADD/ADHD normally have difficulty in at least two of the following four areas of their lives: home, school, social interactions, and work.

Although ADD/ADHD symptoms usually become noticeable in early childhood, unless associated with some type of brain injury, some symptoms, if untreated, may continue into adulthood, posing life-long challenges. Some children with ADD/ADHD may experience a two- to four-year developmental delay that makes them seem less mature and responsible than their peers.

Teens with ADD/ADHD are especially vulnerable since during the teen years academic, social, and organizational demands usually increase.

Many adults with ADD/ADHD were never properly diagnosed as children. As a result, they grew up struggling with a disability they did not even know they had. Others were diagnosed as "hyperactive" and were told their symptoms would disappear as they grew older, but nothing changed because no treatments were applied.

The fact that ADD/ADHD often persists into adulthood has come to light only fairly recently. There has been a belief among professionals for many years that children and adolescents would outgrow their symptoms of ADD/ADHD by puberty, and certainly by adulthood. However, research has shown that as many as 67 percent of children diagnosed with ADD/ADHD will continue to have symptoms of the disorder that interfere with academic, vocational or social functioning during their entire adult lives. Individuals with the disorder can still be successful in life, but without proper treatment, ADD/ADHD can cause serious consequences, including low self-esteem, academic failure, depression, trouble with relationships, career under-achievement and a possible increase in the risk of antisocial and even criminal behavior.

CAUSES OF ADD/ADHD

No single factor has been pinpointed as the cause of ADD/ADHD. In my opinion, genetics may play a role, but the most likely causes include poor nutrition, insufficient sleep, allergies, negative lifestyle habits, environmental pollution and stress. We will be looking at these causes in more detail in later chapters.

TREATMENT

By far the most widespread approach to the treatment of ADD/ADHD in the United States today is drug therapy as a first, and too often the only, step.

I recommend a more balanced and natural approach, focusing on proper nutrition and rest, positive changes in lifestyle, support and encouragement, and the avoidance of toxic environmental factors. Treatment should begin with parental training, professional medical recommendations, education on ADD/ADHD and proper nutrition, individual and family counseling, self-help, natural home treatments and programs and – when and only if required – medication.

I believe with my program than nearly 100 percent of children affected by ADD/ADHD would experience great relief from the symptoms of ADD/ADHD with modest changes in their diet and lifestyle. There are three primary modifications that every patient has responded positively to:

- Healthy diet with appropriate supplementation: conversion from junk foods to wholesome natural foods, including all-natural vitamin supplements, minerals and herbs. If the child is unwilling to make a major shift in dietary habits, you will still begin to see changes by giving them proper supplementation.

- Outdoor activity: balancing a child's time between outdoor physical activities and indoor television and computer-related activities.

- A stable family structure with the objective of minimizing a child's stress. A very valuable first step that brings results is instituting consistent bedtimes and rest times for children.

My balanced treatment approach is detailed in later chapters. You can also visit my website at www.papaschoice.com for specifics.

A boy on two different medications was brought to see me. His teachers complained about his behavior and failure to pay attention. I took his history and found that his parents had been experimenting with different types of nutrition and supplementation. I worked with the mother to add more structure to his diet and switch him to my natural line of supplements that I developed specifically to assist children with symptoms of ADD/ADHD. We began seeing visual results on a daily and weekly basis in school and other activities and within six weeks the boy was off the medications. The parents were happy, but told me they had no time to make additional dietary changes that I knew would result in even greater benefits.

3

HOW DID WE GET HERE?

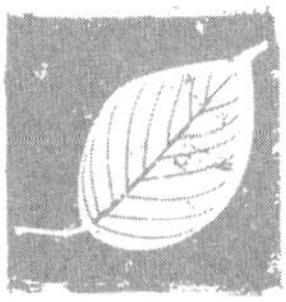

Looking back to my childhood over 40 years ago, I do not recall hearing of friends, family or fellow students having the behavioral or focusing problems experienced by so many American children today. Back then there was no ADD/ADHD "epidemic" like we are experiencing today. Children today are facing many other widespread health problems besides ADD/ADHD, especially those resulting from obesity – including diabetes, the rates of which have skyrocketed in recent years.

Why is this? Why in just a short number of years has our nation become so unhealthy – to the point where the young generation of today is the first since our great nation's inception that is expected to live fewer years than their parents?

When I was a child, we were not allowed to sit in front of the TV after school for hours on end. If we wanted to watch TV for a little while, first we had to finish our homework and have our chores done. Even then, we preferred to go outdoors and play games or sports rather than just fall in front of the TV for endless hours. I remember there were always plenty of outdoor activities available to me.

Today, many things are different. More parental supervision is needed rather than less. Video games and, increasingly, the internet pose serious problems for our children – ranging from obesity caused by lack of physical activity to isolation and difficulties in communicating and, at the extreme end of the scale, losing touch with reality and vulnerability to pedophiles.

Even if a child is allowed to go out and play with friends after school, parents have to worry more about who they are playing with. Are their friends into drugs? Are strangers prowling around? These considerations are more important today than they were 40 years ago.

Also, eating habits and food values have changed drastically over the last 40 years. The snacks I typically got were milk, cookies and fruit. We were not permitted large amounts of sodas, cakes and candies except on special occasions like holidays and birthdays. Today it seems there are endless sugary and greasy snacks available to children throughout the day. The advent of "fast foods" and "quick" meals has created a situation in which sound nutritional choices for children, such as fresh and whole foods, are pushed aside and frequently excluded completely.

I ate a controlled diet growing up. My parents knew what I ate for breakfast, lunch and dinner and made sure I had a good nutritional profile. In those days we had fresh foods, including fruits and vegetables, which were simpler and contained fewer preservatives, artificial ingredients and chemical toxins, such as pesticides and herbicides, than today's foods. Much of the food we ate came from local farmers, who regularly tended to the quality of their soil and did not use pesticides. The food not only tasted better but was fresher and had far more vitamins and nutrients than the manufactured and processed foods eaten so extensively today.

We had structured, predictable times for meals – there was no "eating on the run" such as we have today. Even though our school lunches, outside of the bagged lunches we brought, were not great, they were still better than the school lunch menus at most schools today. These menus are simply advertising campaigns for soda and snack chip corporations.

Growing up, I felt that my activities were well structured, making me feel more secure about my life. There was less stress back then. We were not expected to be "super-achievers." We had school, homework, sports and play. We were required to behave well and do well at school, but there was not too much pressure to achieve extraordinary goals that would drive a child crazy.

Today we expect children to be high-achieving, multi-taskers who have to do a lot just to get through the day. Why do we have such high expectations for our children? There is enormous pressure in childhood – a time when young people should be experiencing unstructured freedom and creativity to discover themselves and develop the higher aspects of cognition and mental capacity. To escape their stress, children reach for television, video games, bad foods and snacks, and other negative choices.

To reverse this trend, parents first need to examine their lifestyle and choices, and the impact of these on the family. It is helpful to do this with an understanding of the larger perspective. Culturally, we have shifted and continue to shift; we are more chaotic and "on the go" today than ever. More women are in the workforce with careers, rather than jobs, making it challenging for parents to provide healthy, home-cooked meals and have family time together. Families are also more fragmented today: Higher divorce rates are resulting in children living between two homes, and both children and parents have many different activities and obligations pulling the family in different directions. Families are also more transient, moving from place to place for new job opportunities. There is an enormous amount of energy required to start anew and rebuild support systems. On top of all this, many have become chronic high-achievers and multi-taskers, expecting so much out of themselves, others and life. We push ourselves, often to the maximum, to secure our place in society, regardless of the impact on our health and the health of our families. We can stop this trend. As parents, we must first take the responsibility to define what is healthy and appropriate for ourselves and our families.

Children can be taught to express their feelings and emotions healthfully and to discriminate between good and bad choices, but only when there is a solid foundation of love, care and respect at home. Children need to be given the freedom to be children when they are meant to be children – at young ages; this will allow them to develop the confidence, intelligence and self-esteem to become well-adjusted adults.

THE SCHOOL ENVIRONMENT

Our public school system seems to have changed considerably since I attended school as a child. Classes today are often overcrowded and there is a tendency for bright children to become bored or slowed down in the midst of large classes designed to make groups of children "conform," limiting the expression of their individual talents and imagination. This may be one reason why drugs are recommended by teachers who find "problem" children in their classes – in other words, children who don't conform. Many of these children, who would excel in supportive environments, are now suffering in another way – as ADD/ADHD patients.

Is the real problem children's failure to conform? Or is it a misguided desire for *uniformity*? It may be that today's schools just want to pass everyone in a uniform manner through the system without consideration of a child's individual talents and tendencies because it is easier for them to do so. How many non-conforming, bored children are diagnosed as hyperactive or ADD/ADHD rather than high-achieving? The majority, I believe. If a child is bored and restless in a class, we should first find a way to challenge that child at a higher level of education rather than blame the child for failing to conform to a potentially boring curriculum.

A young boy's parents once came to see me, concerned about a diagnosis of ADD/ADHD. They didn't want their child on medication. His symptoms were lack of concentration and focus in school, failure to pay attention and fidgeting. I asked his mother: "What does he like to do?" She explained that her son loved to draw. I asked, "Can he draw for 20 minutes? Can he draw for 40 minutes? An hour?" The mother replied, yes, her son was able to sit and draw for an hour, sometimes more. I explained that he probably did not have ADD/ADHD, because he could focus on an activity for this length of time. The difference in this case was that the boy *enjoyed* drawing.

Often, medical professionals and school administrators are too quick to make a diagnosis of ADD/ADHD, when the issue is more related to a child's preferences – likes and dislikes. Culturally, we must evaluate the effectiveness of old classroom paradigms and consider new teaching methods that are a better match for evolving learning styles. Most children today can easily sit quietly and watch videos: This suggests that we need to incorporate more videos and other creative teaching methods that are both engaging and educational. Children today are multi-taskers. At home, they listen to iPods, e-mail their friends, and do their homework, all while engaged with their Playstations. Many kids in the technology generation are brighter than average and are quick to pick up on things; they often require more stimulation and attention than teachers of 40 students can provide on their own.

We need to adjust our educational system to handle more individual needs and educate our children based upon those individual needs, rather than just pushing children into drug programs to make things easier for the school administrators.

Celebrity chef Jamie Oliver was appalled by the unhealthy food being served to British school students and in 2005 began a drive to transform the nutritional quality of school meals. His campaign struck a nerve with the public and gathered such momentum that the UK government intervened, pledging funds to improve the quality of school meals and banish junk food from menus.

At around the same time – May 2005 – The Alliance for a Healthier Generation (a joint initiative of the William J. Clinton Foundation and the American Heart Association) was formed to address the issues that contribute to childhood obesity and to inspire all young Americans to develop lifelong healthy habits. Among its initiatives is a program to assist schools to make available to their students healthier alternatives to high-calorie soft drinks – with the cooperation of leading soft-drinks manufacturers.

If we demand it, we can get schoolteachers involved and start improving our schools' diet programs and activity programs. Children in school can be taught the importance of good sleep, good diet, and balanced activities, including proper exercise and avoidance of too much TV or video games. Schools may say this is the parents' job, but it is also the responsibility of our children's teachers. In fact, is everyone's responsibility to work together: as responsible parents, we need to work closely together with school administrators to create healthy solutions that work for everyone.

Imagine what a good influence it would be for our children to see their parents working with the school to bring more balance into their lives. Don't you agree we would have healthier and better-behaved children? Not only would their jobs be easier, but it would help us too. Why don't we do it? It is up to us to influence our schools and motivate them to implement positive changes. Otherwise, the quality of our school system and our children's education will continue to deteriorate over time.

The Influence Of The Drug Companies

The current situation makes you wonder who is influencing our teachers and school administrators regarding our children's health. Unfortunately, today it is often doctors, psychologists, and especially the pharmaceutical companies who descend on school administrators and teachers. They visit administrators directly or send their representatives to speak and lecture to the teachers individually or in groups about the wonderful effects of drugs – a campaign for controlling our children's behavior and "improving" conditions in school. This is simply scandalous and ought to be a matter for public outrage.

The fact is that drugging our children will not help anyone at the school, including the teachers, and it certainly will not help the parents. The mass distribution of drugs to our children helps only profit-hungry pharmaceutical companies and their friends and associates. Why is it that we believe wholeheartedly what we read, see on television or hear from our children's teachers about the benefits of pharmaceutical drugs? As parents, we need to understand that the pharmaceutical industry is a *business* whose livelihood and that of millions of employees is dependent on the number of people buying their product. They will target every possible audience to satisfy their key objectives of increasing market share and satisfying shareholders. Their marketing campaigns are developed to entice us to want their product, instructing us to "ask your doctor" about the benefits of these drugs.

A 20-minute visit to the doctor is not enough time to properly diagnose your child and put him or her on psychotropic medications that have the possibility of creating another lifetime user.

Informed parents must know that when pharmaceutical companies approach schools they are doing so as a business, with the sole purpose of meeting business objectives. They know that the more children who use and become reliant on these drugs, the more they stand to profit. What happens to our children as a result of taking these drugs is of far less importance and concern. Have we really become so weak that we will allow commercial interests to take over our responsibilities as parents? I don't think so, and I don't believe we will continue to give in to these forces and let ourselves and our children become drug-dependent fools.

It is up to you, as the parent, to be vigilant and careful with your child's health and to take advantage of any and every alternative you can find to dangerous drug therapy, which should always be the last and most desperate of choices.

You can make all the difference by monitoring the diet and lifestyle of your child. Make sure your child has healthy food at every meal, daily routines, consistent rest and sleep, and regular and frequent exercise and you will see excellent results beyond your expectations.

Our children are our future and as we support them we support the development of the future for all.

4

Cause For Concern: The Effects of Ritalin and Other Drugs

Psychostimulants, mind-altering drugs, are the most widely used medications for the management of ADD/ADHD related symptoms. Among these are Ritalin and Concerta (methylphenidate), Dexedrine and Dextrostat (dextroamphetamine or d-amphetamine), Adderall (D-amphetamine and amphetamine mixture), Desoxyn and Gradumet (methamphetamine), and Cylert (pemoline).

These are very powerful drugs whose effects can be even stronger than those of common street drugs like cocaine or methamphetamine (speed). The most common side effects are reduction in appetite and difficulty sleeping. Some children experience "stimulant rebound," periods of negative mood, fatigue, or increased activity when the medication is wearing off. There may be an initial, slight effect on height and weight gain. A detailed survey of these drugs and their effects is provided in the Review of Medication section on page 107.

Ritalin

The most common ADD/ADHD drug treatment among pediatricians and representatives of the mental-health community is methylphenidate (Ritalin, Methylin). Let's look at it closely before considering its use.

First approved by the FDA in 1955, Ritalin had become widely used for behavioral control by the mid-1960s. It is produced by the Swiss-based multinational pharmaceutical company Novartis. According to the Drug Enforcement Administration (DEA), the United States buys and uses 85 percent of the world's Ritalin. A UN agency known as the International Narcotics Control Board, or INCB, reported in 1995 that "10 to 12 percent of all boys between the ages of 6 and 14 in the U.S. have been diagnosed as having ADD [attention-deficit disorder, now referred to as ADD/ADHD] and are being treated with methylphenidate."

Many responsible parents are concerned about evidence they say confirms a close relationship between use of prescribed psychotropic drugs and subsequent use of illegal drugs, including cocaine and heroin. While the United States has spent more than $70 billion on the war on illegal drugs, says Bruce Wiseman, president of the Citizens Commission on Human Rights, a California-based organization that investigates violations of human rights by mental-health practitioners, "If you think the Colombian drug cartel is the biggest drug dealer in the world, think again. It's your neighborhood psychiatrist."

Twenty-eight years ago the World Health Organization (WHO) concluded that Ritalin was pharmacologically similar to cocaine in its pattern of abuse and cited Ritalin as a Schedule II drug – the *most addictive* in medical usage. The Department of Justice followed WHO by citing Ritalin in Schedule II of the Controlled Substances Act as having a very high potential for abuse. As a Schedule II drug, Ritalin joins morphine, opium, cocaine and the heroin substitute methadone.

Eighty-five percent of all the Ritalin produced in the world is used in the United States.

According to a report in the 1995 Archives of General Psychiatry, "Cocaine is one of the most reinforcing and addicting of the abused drugs and has pharmacological actions that are very similar to those of Ritalin." In the same year the DEA also made the Ritalin/cocaine connection, warning that Ritalin "shares many of the pharmacological effects of . . . cocaine . . . Ritalin substitutes for cocaine and d-amphetamine in a number of behavioral paradigms," and expressing concern that "one in every 30 Americans between 5 and 19 years old has a prescription for the drug."

Ritalin is being prescribed to millions of American children. Children's Hospital in Washington has been running television advertisements expressing concern. According to its spokes-woman, Lynn Cantwell, the ads were part of a series covering many medical issues. "We wanted to advocate that children get a comprehensive evaluation because we are finding that children were coming in who were taking Ritalin who actually did not have ADD/ADHD."

Some researchers say that Ritalin does not correct biochemical imbalances and may, in fact, cause them. Is it possible that pediatricians, parents, and teachers are not aware of these potential hazards because a large body of research demonstrating the ill effects of this drug has been ignored or suppressed in order to encourage the sale of the drug?

SIDE EFFECTS OF RITALIN

According to some experts, such as psychiatrist Dr. Peter Breggin, author of *Talking Back to Ritalin*, Ritalin has side effects that are ignored by advocates of the drug. These side effects may include:

- decreased blood flow to the brain, an effect recently shown to be caused by cocaine, where it is associated with impaired thinking ability and memory loss, and may routinely cause other gross malfunctions in the developing brain of the child.

- disruption of growth hormone, leading to suppression of growth in the body and brain.

- permanent neurological tics, including those of Tourette's Syndrome.

- addiction and abuse, including withdrawal reactions on a daily basis.

- psychosis (mania), depression, insomnia, agitation and social withdrawal.

- possible shrinkage (atrophy) or other permanent physical abnormalities in the brain.

- worsening of the very symptoms the drug is supposed to improve, including hyperactivity and inattention.

- decreased ability to learn.

Ritalin and other stimulants are prescribed in the hope of alleviating the inattention, hyperactivity, and impulsiveness shown by ADD/ADHD sufferers. These drugs "work" by producing robotic or zombie-like behavior in children. This enforced docility and seeming obedience can produce a few weeks of subdued behavior but may have no positive effect on academic achievement – and no positive long-term effects at all.

Contrary to claims by drug advocates, giving Ritalin to a child does not help prevent future problems such as school failure or delinquency. Some maintain that a portion of the increased school violence we are seeing these days results from the use of Ritalin and other drugs: Children who may "go off" the medication or not take the medication properly can suffer "reactions" that can prove disastrous to society. This claim is still under investigation, but I believe it has great merit – see the examples in the sidebar later in this chapter.

Needless to say, I do not regard the fact that violence may be committed by children who stop taking the medication without medical supervision, or who do not take it exactly as prescribed, as a reason for putting blame on either the children concerned or their parents. Rather, I regard it as a further reason to avoid putting children onto these drugs wherever possible.

Many experts feel that, as I pointed out in the previous chapter, parents and teachers and even doctors have been badly misled by drug-company marketing practices. Many schoolchildren receiving drugs have been identified by teachers as requiring treatment for ADD/ADHD. In many cases, I believe, these teachers have been misled and misinformed by promotional campaigns designed to support the sale of these drugs as ADD/ADHD medication funded by our government as well as the drug companies.

Are mind-altering drugs ever an appropriate approach to helping our children? Why not look at the natural approach while identifying and meeting the individual needs of the children in our care?

The motto of every parent or teacher who is tempted to resort to the doping of children should be, "First educate, don't medicate."

THE CHEMISTRY OF VIOLENT CHILDREN

Violent acts at schools across the nation, like those at Columbine High School, have been committed by children receiving psychiatric care, counseling, and drugs such as Ritalin. Some organizations, such as The Citizens Commission on Human Rights, claim that the over-use of Ritalin is at least partly to blame for the escalating incidents of children committing acts of violence upon other children. They claim the problem has reached pandemic proportions and will get worse before it gets better. Other experts place the blame on inadequate parenting, while legislators propose new laws.

Some experts claim drugs like Ritalin can cause psychotic reactions resulting in violent behavior toward others and even feelings of suicide. Defenders of the drug claim those reactions are symptoms of the condition, not the drug itself. Support for the claim that the use of Ritalin can cause psychotic reactions can be found in medical literature and studies. There are many medically credible documents and references available listing a large number of warnings and side effects to the drug.

"The use of Ritalin on children has no purpose other than to slow them down, shut them up, and make it more difficult for them to move around," says Dennis H. Clarke, Chairman, Executive Advisory Board, Citizens Commission On Human Rights International. He believes that Ritalin is an easy way out for parents and teachers, rather than dealing directly with behavior problems in children. Clarke claims that children who take Ritalin in elementary school are often switched to Prozac and other drugs as they grow older. The effects of Ritalin can cause problems long after the prescription is stopped, he added. "When they go through puberty, this becomes true speed," explained Clarke. "They get these flashbacks and their

"Utah is reported to have the highest per capita use of Ritalin in the nation. A call to a local elementary school found a teacher who believes strongly in the use of the drug to control otherwise difficult children. She did not want her name published, but confirmed that she routinely makes recommendations for children in her classes to be given the drug. All the children she has recommended have ended up with the prescription, and their parents have expressed gratitude. She said 11 of the 29 children in her first-grade class are now taking the drug in school each day." – WorldNetDaily

[July 2002, http://www.worldnetdaily.com/search.asp]

thinking goes out of control. They're now looking for downers. They want the anti-depressants. They want the tranquilizer."

Dr. Ann Blake Tracy, director of the International Coalition for Drug Awareness, is equally concerned. "They are switching lots of these kids from Ritalin to Prozac – the frying pan into the fire routine" (www.WorldNetDaily.com). She also points out that adults who use such drugs also commit violent crimes at a higher rate. Dr. Tracy is from Utah, where the use of Ritalin and Prozac are reported to be at a rate three times greater than the rest of the country per capita. She notes that Utah's rate of murders and suicides has also increased by a similar amount.

There have been numerous incidents in which young children have brought weapons to school. Young children have recently held students at bay with guns at schools in Utah and Idaho. Some have used them, and one incident in Arkansas brought international attention when four school children and one teacher were shot dead at a middle school.

Shouldn't we consider the possibility that drugging our children is making them more violent?

Teachers, school administrators, and even doctors hold to the belief that if a child responds well to Ritalin, then it is safe to conclude that the child suffers from ADD/ADHD. Does that make sense? In my view, allowing the positive response to a drug to determine a diagnosis is utterly nonsensical – backwards medicine. It's a little like giving a sleeping pill to a child and, when the child sleeps longer than usual, concluding that she must have been suffering from insomnia! Except, of course, that Ritalin is much more dangerous than a sleeping pill.

The Hippocratic oath that all doctors take upon successfully completing their requirements says: First do no harm. This is why the process of medicine since Hippocrates' time has been diagnose first, administer second. In addition to the obligation placed upon them by the Hippocratic Oath, I believe that physicians have a moral obligation to take the time to consider a child's individual situation and health profile before manipulating him or her with medication.

Luvox, a cousin of Prozac, has been approved by the FDA for pediatric use, although research shows that a small percentage of patients experience adverse effects such as mania, bouts of irritability, aggression and hostility. But many physicians still prescribe it to children.

"Warning: sufficient data on the safety and efficacy (effectiveness) of long-term use of Ritalin in children are not yet available," warns Novartis in a product information release. The warning is intended to serve as a protection from liability. The drug has been on the market for 50 years.

"In other words," say Clarke "if you have a child on Ritalin, and leave the child on for a 'long term,' which is not defined but can be assumed to mean over three weeks, you are on your own as far as Novartis is concerned. They have warned you."

Herbert S. Okun, a member of the International Drug Control Board for the United Nations, held a news conference to issue a warning. He said his board is very concerned that Ritalin is greatly over-prescribed in the U.S. He said there are 330 million daily doses of Ritalin taken each day in the U.S., compared with just 65 million for the rest of the world.

Consumption of prescription antidepressants by children has skyrocketed – currently growing at annual rate of nine percent. Are all of these kids really depressed or handicapped? Or are they simply malnourished? Did you ever notice that our kids consume massive amounts of processed foods, fast foods, junk foods with added sugars? Our young children and teenagers have some of the worst diets anywhere on the planet – diets that are altering the natural balance of chemicals in their brains. Rather than prescribing good nutrition and exercise habits, many doctors prescribe yet more chemicals that only mask the symptoms. Maybe what the kids need is real food rather than more drugs that can make them violent, indifferent and suicidal.

Parents Kept In The Dark?

Many parents are not offered any alternatives other than a prescription drug for their children with ADD/ADHD. The parent may be told that a child's grades will suffer or continue to suffer unless the child is put on Ritalin. Most parents just accept this without question. Even the manufacturer of Ritalin makes no claim that the drug has ever improved a child's ability to learn or retain information.

As parents, we must be careful to investigate alternatives prior to subscribing to and administering a drug that we know has harmful effects. Ritalin is not a "smart pill" – it is actually a "dumb pill" for the many children who don't need it. A better report card for the long term will never come from drugging, but only from naturally occurring improvements in our children's mental, emotional and physical health through better food, better food supplements, proper sleep, better daily routines and better parenting.

Few Americans are aware of how many children involved in shooting incidents are among those taking mind-altering drugs prescribed for ADD/ADHD or other alleged mental illnesses. The slaughter at Columbine High School became a national wake-up call. Not many in the mental-health community have been willing to talk about the possibility that heavily prescribed drugs and related violence may be linked. Those who try to investigate will learn that almost all data concerning violence and psychotropic drugs are protected by the confidentiality that is provided to minors. Well, that's fine, but let's not be unreasonable and ignore the relationship of violence and drugs. To many of us the connection is clear, no matter how much anyone tries to cover it up.

Here are a few cases of children on prescription drugs that illustrate the obvious relationship to violence:

Shawn Cooper, a 15-year-old sophomore at Notus Junior-Senior High School in Notus, Idaho, was taking Ritalin, the most commonly prescribed stimulant, for bipolar disorder when he fired two shotgun rounds, narrowly missing students and school staff.

Eric Harris, an 18-year-old senior at Columbine High School in Littleton, Colorado, killed a dozen students and a teacher before taking his own life. An autopsy on Harris showed that at the time of his death his body contained a "therapeutic" level of Luvox, one of the new selective serotonin reuptake inhibitor, or SSRI, antidepressants approved in 1997 by the Food and Drug Administration, or FDA, for children up to the age of 17 for treatment of obsessive-compulsive disorder (OCD).

T.J. Solomon, a 15-year-old at Heritage High School in Conyers, Georgia, was being treated with Ritalin for depression when he opened fire on and wounded six of his classmates.

Kip Kinkel, a 15-year-old at Thurston High School in Springfield, Oregon, murdered his parents and then proceeded to school where he opened fire on students in the cafeteria, killing two and wounding 22. Kinkel had been prescribed both Ritalin and Prozac.

Mitchell Johnson, 13, and Andrew Golden, 11, opened fire on their classmates at Westside Middle School in Jonesboro, Arkansas. Johnson had been receiving psychiatric counseling and, although information about the psychotropic drugs that may have been prescribed for him has not been made public, his attorney, Val Price, responded when asked about it: "I think that is confidential information, and I don't want to reveal that."

These and other examples have been written about and seen on TV over the years, yet few people are making the connection between these children, the drugs they take and the violence they commit.

GETTING YOUR CHILD OFF RITALIN AND OTHER ADD/ADHD MEDICATION

You may have found much of the information presented in this chapter shocking, and even frightening – and rightly so. But you may have found it particularly worrisome if your child, or the children of your friends and relatives, are taking Ritalin or other drugs for ADD/ADHD.

Do not panic. It is extremely unlikely that your child will commit violence of the kind described above, or of a lesser kind. After all, up to six million American children are taking Ritalin and other drugs for ADD/ADHD, and school shootings are still rare occurrences.

Under no circumstances should you stop your child's medication without first discussing the matter with a knowledgeable and experienced health professional. Stopping the medication can lead to serious withdrawal reactions, and you and your child need to be aware of the possibilities of such reactions, and to be under professional supervision.

Continue to have your child take the medication exactly as prescribed until you have consulted your doctor or health professional, and then take only the steps he or she recommends.

5 A Natural Approach: Getting Started?

Children with ADD/ADHD risk facing serious problems in the future, including academic underachievement, difficulty with peers, and problems with authority. As many as 67 percent of childhood sufferers continue to experience symptoms of ADD/ADHD in adulthood. Early identification of the condition along with treatment is necessary to protect our children and young adults and prevent them from the dangers of premature labeling and treatment protocols issued by those who are ill-prepared to help them over the long run.

We don't have to blame ourselves as parents, but we do have to take positive actions to protect our children in the most natural and safe manner possible. Life with an ADD/ADHD child can be challenging and it is important to remember that children with ADD/ADHD can and do succeed with our help.

SHOP AROUND FOR PROFESSIONAL HELP

Many of our health care providers treat ADD/ADHD children and adults with drug therapies, psychological and psychiatric therapies, stress reduction therapies, and in some extreme cases confinement, hospitalization, and institutionalization, which may end in the banishment of the child or adult from normal society.

Before accepting advice from a health professional, ask them questions related to the diagnosis and treatment of ADD/ADHD.

- How many of their clients have the disorder?
- What methods will they use to evaluate the child?
- What types of treatment do they support?
- What kind of success rate do they have?
- Do they have a natural approach program that does not include the regular drug medications most often recommended?

You must be your child's best advocate and protect his or her best interests. I do not recommend jumping on a drug medication program unless it is an emergency situation. Why should you take the risk of drug side effects including long-term complications and other problems if it is not warranted? You and your child have the right to establish a natural, non-invasive, and non-drug treatment program for a permanent healthy solution to ADD/ADHD conditions.

Fortunately, there are a growing number of health professionals who recognize the relationship of ADD/ADHD symptoms to diet, environment, daily activities, and especially to nutritional deficiencies. There are still too few such professionals, but if you look around you can find one.

Remember that health begins at home. There is nothing wrong with beginning a natural and self-reliant approach to the problem at home. Self-help is a tried and true American tradition! Unless you regard your child's condition as an emergency situation requiring immediate outside help, begin with the recommendations I make in the remainder of this chapter and the following chapters.

Behavioral training is important for children who have ADD/ADHD. Problem solving, communication, and self-advocacy skills, as well as positive reinforcement, are especially helpful for teenagers. All of these things can be considered to improve symptoms of ADD/ADHD.

The behavioral approach at home with children should include an effective discipline system. Let me stress that when I say "discipline" I do not mean punishment! True discipline is a way of helping children to learn appropriate behavior – to acquire *self*-discipline. There are programs to help you learn proactive parenting methods such as STEP (Systematic Training for Effective Parenting). See Resource Section on page 115 for information on how to acquire this program.

You can assist your children with social issues such as teaching them to make friends and working with others. Most importantly, you can identify your child's gifts and abilities and build on them until your child feels a sense of accomplishment. Set up "quality time" with your child and offer positive reinforcement that will strengthen your child's self-worth.

You must offer your unconditional love and your child will respond positively.

Let's review some natural approach recommendations as related to children with ADD/ADHD:

1. Parental kindness including love, encouragement and approval.

2. Less television and video games, more outdoor activities.

3. Avoidance of potential environmental allergens and pollutants such as tobacco smoke, radiation, etc.

4. Avoidance of emotional stress.

5. Good nutrition. Regular meals with fresh foods including fruits, grains, and vegetables. Plenty of fluids. Avoidance of "ziggies" (chemical or synthetic sources of food additives, colors, flavors, preservatives and stimulants). Avoidance of excessive amounts of refined sugar, refined flour, chocolates, sweetened sodas, fried foods and hydrogenated fats.

6. Regular routines of sleep, bathing, hygiene, play, exercise and learning.

7. Nutritional food supplements. Regular appropriate pure vitamin/mineral nutritional dietary supplementation and/or herbal supplementation without yeast or excessive excipients (additives such as sweeteners, fillers, binders, coatings, flavors and preservatives).

Most of the above recommendations are appropriate for adults, as well. The most important ones, in my view, are a good, nutritious diet, and nutritional and herbal supplements. I will deal more with the question of diet and supplements in Chapters 6,7 and 8.

ASKING THE RIGHT QUESTIONS

No one knows your child as well as you do and the parent is always the best source of information about the child.

If you believe that your child has an ADD/ADHD condition, then asking yourself and your child the right questions will get you started on the best path to helping them. Don't assume that anyone else can provide answers you are not able to find yourself. It is not always easy, but taking the time to be observant and using your instincts and natural detective skills will often provide you with answers that no therapist, doctor, teacher or other professional can give you.

In my opinion, physicians should be required to take a full *lifestyle* history, in addition to a medical history, of each and every child whom they suspect of having ADD/ADHD. In one case, a mother came to me not knowing where to start. The school had called suggesting that her child be put onto medication for ADD/ADHD because half her child's teachers were complaining about her behavior. I took a full lifestyle history, examining this child's patterns, from morning through sleep time, and discovered that she was not only skipping breakfast but consuming only soda an junk food for lunch. I immediately made the

recommendation to begin by stabilizing the diet. The mother agreed to daily breakfasts, and decided that a bag lunch would be far more suitable than financing the unhealthy choices that her child was making. She also agreed to add my supplements. Within just a couple of weeks, her child's behavior had stabilized.

When medical practitioners are willing to look at the whole picture and ask the right questions, they will often uncover simple answers to seemingly complex issues. It is our responsibility as parents and practitioners to ask the right questions so that we can address the core cause of illness and disease.

To get started, ask yourself the following questions and when necessary interview your child, writing down the answers.

NUTRITION

What are you feeding your child? And what else is your child eating and drinking?

Take your time and find out what your child is eating on a daily basis. List and break down his diet into amounts, times fed and most important, the contents of his meals, such as breakfast, lunch, and dinner. Also, include specifics about snacks and beverages taken throughout the day.

I have found that putting a child on a proper diet is *at least* half the solution to problems of ADD/ADHD. Children should eat fresh, healthy foods and avoid excessive amounts of sugars (from sodas, cereals, candy, and so on). They should never eat treats or other foods containing artificial colors, preservatives, or synthetic ingredients. Whenever possible, I recommend organic foods free of chemicals and Genetically Modified Organisms (GMOs) – plants or animals (or products thereof) whose genetic makeup has been determined or altered by genetic engineering. I will look at diet and nutrition in greater detail in a later chapter, but these are the initial diet factors to be aware of.

FOOD CRAVINGS

What snacks does your child crave or ask for?

If your child constantly asks for certain treats, for example a chocolate this or that, or something else, this may give you an idea of something she should avoid – especially if you notice that she becomes fussy or difficult shortly after getting it. You can replace unhealthy snacks and treats with healthy ones. For example, if your daughter reacts badly to chocolate but insists on chocolate things, you can offer her some sliced fruit or another healthy "sweet" that does not cause a negative reaction. Eventually she will be glad to have it and even request the new, healthier "treat" from you.

SLEEP

What are your child's sleeping habits? At what times does he go to bed? How many times does he wake up during the night? How many hours a day does he sleep? Does he take naps? Where does he sleep? What position does he normally sleep in? Is his mattress old or uncomfortable? Does he have a pleasant place to sleep in that is quiet and friendly?

Lack of sleep is a primary contributing factor to hyperactivity, and cumulative lack of sleep leads to the worst of ADD/ADHD symptoms. The importance of regular rest and sleep for your child's health cannot be overemphasized. You can give your child a calming herbal tea at bedtime, or some warm milk, or a natural, botanical sleep aid when necessary to help prepare your child for a deep and refreshing sleep. A calming and relaxing nightly ritual prior to bed that includes reading or soft music can help too.

TV, VIDEO GAMES AND COMPUTERS

How many hours a day does your child spend watching TV, playing video games, working on the computer or playing on the computer?

If your child is straining her nervous system with excess TV, video games or computer viewing, this has to stop. If these activities are not limited, even a normally sensitive child can develop nervous disorders. For an ADD/ADHD child or adult, it is vital that these activities be severely curtailed or eliminated.

EXERCISE

What physical activities such as sports or exercise does your child participate in on a daily basis?

Daily exercise, especially structured exercise such as supervised individual or team sports, is essential for the normal physical development and health of your child. This is true not only for physical health but also for mental and emotional health. Exercising in groups provides peer support, bonding and confidence through cooperation and learning.

ALLERGIES

Does your child have any allergies? Also, what environmental toxins is your child exposed to on a daily basis?

If you know your child has certain food or environmental allergies then, of course, you can take steps to make sure your child is protected from these allergens to the best of your ability. If you don't know, but suspect your child might have allergies to certain foods like wheat, milk, peanuts, soy, shellfish or environmental allergens like pollen, trees, gasoline, detergents, moldy ventilations, etc., then have your child tested by a health professional who is an expert in allergies to determine any specific allergies your child may have. Specific allergies of any kind may contribute heavily to ADD/ADHD symptoms in children and must be avoided.

POSITIVE AND NEGATIVE INFLUENCES

What are the positive influences on your child? What are the negative influences?

These questions may appear simplistic, but if you think carefully about them, and write down a list of the positive and negative influences on your child, you will be surprised at how much this exercise will help you to get a full picture of your child's life. You will then be able to take steps to accentuate the positive influences in your child's life and eliminate the negative ones. For example, do the parents fight in front of the child? Even if they do not fight openly, are there constant strains and tension in the relationship between the parents? Are punishments too severe? Does your child play with children who are an unhealthy influence on him? Who are your child's friends and who does the child respect and look up to?

HOME SCHEDULE

What is your child's daily schedule? What does she like to do when you are not around to watch her? How does she talk to others on the telephone or during normal interactions?

The daily schedule should be structured and not left up to chance. This is especially important for ADD/ADHD children, who do better when every minute of their daily activity is strictly accounted for.

SCHOOL SCHEDULE

What is your child's school schedule like? What classes during the day does he do well in and which ones is he failing? When he has a great day and feels positive and happy, where is he and what is he doing? Does he do better or worse when he is out of the house on extended vacations, or at camp, or at relatives' homes?

If you find that your child has trouble in classes after lunchtime, you should check his lunch diet and the quality of the food he is eating to see if there is any relationship. If he does better outside the home environment, why?

FAVORITE ACTIVITIES

What activities does your child like; which ones does she dislike?

Does your child have structured activities such as after-school soccer practice or dancing, or something else? Does she follow the scheduled activities without argument and look forward to them? If she has fun doing these activities then all is well, but if she doesn't want to exercise, or has some problems following a schedule of activities, then you need to know why.

ENVIRONMENTAL TOXINS

What environmental toxins and pollutants is your child exposed to at home, at school, and in other places he regularly spends time?

Secondhand tobacco smoke, fumes from glues, paints and varnishes, vehicle exhausts, and many other toxic substances that abound in modern homes and buildings may be seriously affecting your child's mental functioning. See the Resource section on page 115 for some books that can help you evaluate whether you need to make changes in your home or living situation.

Here's an example from my own practice. A mother brought her young boy to me. He was lethargic, not attentive in class and receiving poor grades. She knew that he was not

ADD/ADHD. After inquiring about his routines, we discovered that on the bus journeys both to and from school, he was sitting with his friends in the back of the bus. The windows of the bus were almost always open, causing exhaust gases to circulate around the back of the bus. I asked her to try an experiment and get him to sit in the front of the bus. Almost immediately they noticed more energy and vitality, and within weeks his level of attention in class had improved significantly.

The above questions represent some basic inquiries to help to you analyze and determine positive diet and lifestyles for your child. You don't have to stop here. Think of any further questions or inquires about your child's diet, lifestyle or environment that will help you to improve your child's circumstances and limit the aggravation of your child's ADD/ADHD symptoms. The first step is to determine the best actions to take to help improve your child's daily routine including diet and general lifestyle. After this you can make more natural refinements, adjustments and improvements as you observe your child's development over time. Nor is this questionnaire a replacement for medical opinions from qualified health practitioners.

Here's another example of how taking the time to ask the right questions can make all the difference. The mother of an 8-year-old came to me, saying that her daughter was having trouble sleeping. She slept poorly at best, her grades were suffering and she had trouble paying attention in school. She had bouts of tiredness offset with bouts of hyperactivity. After conducting a full lifestyle history and asking detailed questions over the next week and a half, I discovered that the girl's father was a painter. Her mother explained that at the end of the day he came home through the garage and piled his laundry on the floor right next to the child's room. I immediately suggested a different drop zone for the clothing. In addition, I recommended supplementation, both my multiple vitamins and an anti-oxidant to address the toxic effects of the paint fumes, and having the child drink more water to flush her system. Within a few short weeks, she had recovered and was sleeping soundly.

When a problem arises, pause and take a look at what is happening around you and ask these questions: Is there anything occurring now that wasn't before the problem set in? Are there any allergens (plants, molds, grasses, chemicals, pets etc.) that could be contributing to the problem? What has my child been eating? Have any patterns been disrupted? Asking smart questions is the first place to begin. With these answers, you are not only empowered to understand the reasons of your child's illness, but also to take the proper steps to correct them.

IT'S A FAMILY MATTER

Here is a final, but very important, note to conclude this chapter. My work with ADD/ADHD children and their parents has shown me that in most cases a complete solution to a child's symptoms and problematic behavior cannot be achieved by focusing on the child alone. As the questions I sketched out above will show, many of the primary contributing factors to your child's ADD/ADHD problem may be found in the home. In a very real sense, you, the parents, are part of the problem – and must therefore also be part of the solution.

In addition to the questionnaire you complete for your child, take the time to ask yourself some searching questions. If you find it hard to answer them objectively, ask a close friend or family member for their candid opinion.

Is your own lifestyle or working life too busy, too fast-paced, to allow you to devote sufficient time to your children? Are you under chronic emotional stress because of pressures in your work or financial worries? Any stress you suffer is bound to communicate itself to your children.

Is your relationship with your spouse or partner, and with other members of your family, harmonious, cordial and peaceful? Or tense, strained, and full of unresolved issues and resentments? Your children, consciously or otherwise, may well be acting out *your* tensions.

Do you look after your own nutrition – eat healthy meals, drink plenty of pure water, and avoid junk food, tobacco and immoderate alcohol consumption? If not, it may not be realistic to expect that your children will agree to a different regime.

As I said earlier, we don't need to blame ourselves as parents, but we do need to open our minds to the possibility that changes in our *own* behavior, lifestyle and living conditions may be required! I recognize that this can be a very challenging issue to face, and you may need outside help in rethinking your priorities or reorganizing your life to bring your children back into the center of your and your spouse's life. I urge you, for your children's sake, to take the time to reflect on these aspects, talk them over with your spouse, and seek professional guidance and counseling if needed.

Here again, the Resources section on page 115 lists several resources that can help you explore how to affect positive changes for you and your child.

6
PROPER DIET

I believe that fully half the battle to reduce ADD/ADHD symptoms and manifestations can be won by paying proper attention to diet. Without good, natural, and healthy foods, no one can function properly – much less live up to their potential. Healthy, natural foods are especially important for ADD/ADHD kids and adults who may tend to be, in my experience, especially sensitive to poor diet choices. The first consideration is elimination of toxic substances from the diet. What do I mean by toxic substances? I mean synthetic, chemical food additives and synthetic food fortifications of all types. Here is a short list of toxic substances and food products to avoid in the diet:

- Artificial food colorings and flavorings of any kind
- MSG and other artificial food flavor "enhancers"
- Added yeasts or algae (single-celled bacteria)
- Preservatives such as BHT (butylated hydroxytoluene) and others
- Junk foods (fast foods and most sweets and things in plastic or cellophane wrappers)
- Junk juices – mainly "fruit beverages" that masquerade as fruit juice but are mostly sugar. (Even 100 percent fruit juices should be diluted with pure water, since otherwise their sugar content is likely to be excessively high)

- Sodas (all)
- Sugars (all refined or added sugars)
- Chocolate
- NutraSweet, aspartame-containing sweeteners and all other artificial sweeteners
- Processed meats
- Fried foods
- Chewing gum
- Coffee
- Saturated fats and bad oils (margarine, cotton seed oil, canola oil, safflower oil and any fake oils or fats such as olestra)

At the top of my list are artificial flavors and colors – some of the main culprits. How do you avoid these in foods? The best way is to read the label on the food product. If anything looks suspicious on the label or you have a doubt, then avoid it. Many specialty candy, gum, and "snack" foods contain these artificial toxic ingredients and they should all be avoided. There are plenty of natural treats and snacks like cheese sticks or fresh fruits that can replace these toxic foods and treats. Protect yourself by starting to read all the labels on foods and snacks. You may be surprised by what you learn. A list of additives, including ones that have been banned, is contained in Chapter 8.

Fresh raw organic foods like salads and fruits, steamed vegetables and other "fresh" foods are a critical priority for the ADD/ADHD diet. We need to give fresh organically grown foods in well-balanced meals to our children rather than "dead" meals from Genetically Modified foods in microwave packages and other "dead" canned or packaged foods or those "special" school lunches with no real nutritional value. More fresh food and less dead food is the rule. The body requires the naturally occurring vitamins, minerals, enzymes, and other living bioactive factors found in fresh organic foods in order for us and our children to stay healthy and alert. In addition, non-organic food may contain high levels of residues of pesticides, and even, in animal products, hormones and antibiotics.

Some fresh fruit and vegetables along with lightly cooked grains are essential for our daily diet and the daily diets of our children. Without a proper diet including fresh foods we cannot be healthy nor can we expect our children to be healthy. To be safe, I would also recommend a daily natural multiple vitamin and mineral food supplement for all parents and children with ADD/ADHD. Please note that most multiple supplements contain synthetic vitamins and/or nutrients and should be avoided. The best daily multiple supplements are those that have "naturally occurring" nutrients, with potencies indicated on their labels. (See the Resources section, page 115, for additional resources or visit www.papaschoice.com.)

A proper daily diet with real, natural supplementation goes a long way to help prevent ADD/ADHD symptoms, which are aggravated by toxic snacks and a poor diet lacking in nutritional elements.

In general, meals should be made with fresh ingredients whenever possible. The less processed, the better. Use plenty of fresh vegetables and fruits.

We should also avoid poor diet food choices like hydrogenated fats, fast foods, refined sugars and refined flours. Better to replace these with good fats like fresh, green olive oil, whole, organic, well-prepared fresh meals, raw sugars, and organic whole grain flours. Again, read the labels to help you avoid unnatural and toxic ingredients.

THE IMPORTANCE OF GOOD DIGESTION

Good digestion is vital for health. No matter how good your diet is, or how many toxins you avoid, if you are not digesting your food properly you will not get the essential nutrition that you require for your health. Good digestion means good assimilation of food for the purpose of extracting the essential nutrients that the body requires for good health. This can only happen if the digestive system is functioning properly. Many of our children and their parents have poor digestion due to many years of poor diet and other factors, including parasites. It may surprise you to know that many people have parasites that interfere with proper digestion and have no clue about this. Because we have become a society that ingests large amounts of "dead" foods out of cans and from fast-food establishments or foods "nuked" in microwaves, we are often missing the natural intestinal flora that we used to take for granted. Good bacteria, also known as "intestinal flora," are necessary for a healthy digestive system and for the proper digestion of our foods. These "friendly" bacteria help us to break down the proteins, carbohydrates, and other elements of our food for proper digestion and assimilation of nutrients contained in our foods. Without them we cannot have good digestive function or good health.

I recommend the initial removal of parasites and the addition of "friendly" intestinal bacteria as two initial methods to cleanse our digestive tracts and improve our digestive processes. If you have never done this for yourself or your children, you should do it now. These two approaches for better digestive functioning will go a long way to improve your general health. Combined with the right diet recommended above, these approaches to better digestion should greatly help to reduce ADD/ADHD symptoms and conditions.

The best and most non-invasive way that I know of to remove parasites is to use a natural herbal parasite remedy. These are readily available from your health professional or natural-foods retailer. If you believe that you or your child has a serious parasite infestation, then you should immediately consult with your health professional for specific advice and treatment.

Replenishing and revitalizing your intestinal flora is fairly simple and there are many good natural intestinal protection products and formulas available. Sometimes these products are known as "probiotics" formulations that contain the friendly bacteria we need for good digestive health.

RESTORING THE DIETARY pH BALANCE

Good quality healthy food is the foundation of any diet. One aspect of healthy foods and diet that is overlooked by many is the alkalinity or acidity of foods.

Over the years the American diet and that of the industrialized world has become more acidic. Eating more processed foods, which are generally acidic, and fewer fresh fruits and vegetables, which are generally alkalinizing, tends to increase general acidity of the body. Excess acidity has been associated with lack of energy, poor immune response, and general poor health.

Not everyone agrees with the concept of keeping the diet mainly alkaline, especially our contemporary health professionals who have had no training in this area. But the majority of naturopathic physicians, medical doctors trained in natural nutrition and nutritionists consider an alkaline diet to be crucial for optimal health and prevention of disease. In my experience, alkaline foods help to maintain an alkaline body that is stronger, healthier and more resistant to disease.

The normal, healthy pH or alkaline/acid level of a healthy human is around 7.4 (pH), which means that our body is supposed to be slightly alkaline. Eating more alkaline foods and avoiding more acid-producing foods will help to keep your pH in balance. This diet practice, in my experience, is vital and very helpful for ADD/ADHD persons and goes a long way to prevent symptoms and maintain general good health and focus. If you suspect you are too acidic or have acidic symptoms and would like to find out if your or your child's pH are normal, you can contact your health professional for a test to determine your pH levels.

Some Recommended Alkalizing Foods

Fresh and raw vegetables	Greens: broccoli, Brussels sprouts, cabbage, cauliflower, collard greens, kale Root vegetables: beets, carrots, sweet potatoes, turnips Salad greens: celery, endive, lettuce, parsley, watercress Cucumber, zucchini Green beans and peas Bell peppers, tomatoes Sea vegetables Sprouted vegetables of all types
Fresh fruits	Bananas (excellent!), coconut, grapefruit, lemon, lime
Dried beans and legumes	Lima beans, soy beans, white beans. Slightly alkaline: lentils, tofu.

Nuts and seeds	Pumpkin seeds, sunflower seeds, almonds, sesame seeds, black olives preserved in oil, Brazil nuts, chestnuts
Cold-pressed oils	Coconut oil, cod liver oil, evening primrose oil, olive oil
Nondairy beverages	Almond milk
Dried fruits	Dates, raisins (not those with an acidic taste, such as apricots, apples, pineapple)
Dairy products	Goat's milk products (cheese is mostly acidic – use only moderately) Cow's milk products: large-curd cottage cheese, cream, butter
Grains	Buckwheat, quinoa, spelt
Avocado	
Spices and condiments	Cayenne, red chili pepper, sea salt, stevia. Many fresh or dried herbs and spices are moderately alkaline.

Substantially acidic foods (use moderately or avoid completely)

Meats	Beef, chicken, duck, eggs, gelatin, lobster, pork, seafood
Fatty fish	Salmon, carp, herring, mackerel
Crustaceans	Lobster, shrimp, mussels
Grains	Barley, corn, rye. White rice (use organic brown rice and moderate amounts of organic white rice instead)

Dried beans and legumes	Black beans, kidney beans, red beans, garbanzos (chickpeas)
Mushrooms	
Fruits	Cantaloupe, apple, apricot, all berries, figs (fresh), grape, honeydew, mango, orange, papaya, peach, persimmon, pineapple, tangerine, watermelon
Nuts and seeds	Brazil nuts, flaxseeds, hazelnuts, pecans, walnuts, cashews, peanuts, pistachios.
Oils and fats	Corn oil, hydrogenated oils, margarine, lard
Spices and condiments	Ketchup, mayonnaise, table salt, jam, mustard, soy sauce, vinegar, white sugar, aspartame, molasses, sugar cane, barley malt syrup, maple syrup, yeast.
Refined flour products	White bread, pasta (use non-GMO, organic whole grain flour products instead)
Refined sugars	Both white and brown refined sugars
Refined-sugar-saturated snacks and desserts	Sugary breakfast cereals, cakes, pies, cookies, packed and processed sweet snacks, popcorn
Dairy products	Milk, aged cheese
Condiments	Capers, pickles, pimentos, mustard, ketchup, mayonnaise, excess salt, vinegar
Beverages	Coffee, tea, chocolate milk, sodas, tomato juice, orange juice, grapefruit juice
Alcohol	
Tobacco	

All foods should be eaten in moderation and any foods that produce allergic reactions must be avoided.

An alkaline diet is composed of approximately 75-80 percent alkaline foods and 20-25 percent acid foods.

A WORD ABOUT OILS

Oils and fats are important nutrient foods that we need to eat every day. My general rule about fats and oils is that you should use the best quality available, preferably organic, and that they should be derived from a natural *food* source that you would normally eat. In other words, if the oil comes from a non-food or non-edible source then don't use it.

For example, olive oil, corn oil, sunflower oil, and butter come from natural food sources, which are foods that you would normally eat, but canola oil (from rapeseeds), cottonseed oil (from cotton seeds) and safflower oil (from safflowers) represent oils from non-foods or foods that you normally would not eat. In my opinion, oils derived from non-foods or foods that are not normally eaten are toxic and should be avoided.

Canola oil (rapeseed oil) was originally used as machinery oil 150 years ago and never as a food. There is no tradition that supports the use of canola. It has low amounts of saturated fats, but so does crude petroleum oil, for that matter. Should we be eating petroleum oil? Of course not! In fact, there are traditional references that warn against the use of canola oil. It is very cheap and popular oil these days and found in many food products, but that does not mean it is healthy. I recommend avoiding it.

Water

Pure water is extremely important for your health. Avoid ingesting toxic tap water. You and your children should drink plenty of pure water on a daily basis. Bottled water is fine, but I recommend a water filter that attaches to the kitchen faucet or is installed under your sink. A good filter removes chemicals such as chlorine and other pollutants from your tap water. You can save money on bottled water by filling up containers of cleansed filtered water and storing them for drinking. Use glass containers, because plastic bottles release harmful chemicals into the water. The filter also allows you to use good water for cooking and making beverages.

Synthetic Fragrances And other Environmental Toxins

Fragrance chemicals are compounds that volatilize, or vaporize into the air – that's why we can smell them. They are added to products to give them a scent or to mask the odor of other bad-smelling ingredients. The volatile organic chemicals (VOCs) emitted by fragrance products can contribute to poor indoor air quality and are associated with a variety of adverse health effects. Exposure to fragrance chemicals can cause headaches, eye, nose, and throat irritation, rashes, hyperpigmentation of the skin, nausea, vomiting, coughing, forgetfulness, loss of coordination, dizziness, and other respiratory and/or neurotoxic symptoms. Many fragrance ingredients are respiratory irritants and sensitizers, which can trigger asthma attacks and aggravate sinus conditions. Typically these chemicals are identified by the word "fragrance" on the label.

Of course, as I mentioned in the previous chapter, there are other toxins and chemicals in the environment that should be especially avoided by ADD/ADHD children, including secondhand smoke, chemical pesticides and certain household chemicals. All potential environmental toxins should be separated from children at all times.

6
Nutritional And Herbal Support

Nutritional Support

The importance of proper nutritional support for those with ADD/ADHD *cannot* be overemphasized. Vitamins and minerals for general health are important. This includes vitamin A, C and E (antioxidants). Nutrients that may be helpful in the treatment of hyperactivity and neurological conditions include: vitamin B_1, B_2, B_3, B_6, B_{12}, vitamin C, pantothenic acid, zinc, GABA and others including amino acids such as Taurine and RNA. Visit my website www.papaschoice.com for more information.

Nutritional herbs are also important. The herb *Bacopa monnieria* has been used traditionally as a mental revitalizer and there is clinical evidence that Bacopa can enhance the mental functioning of students. Bacopa is also been used traditionally as an anti-anxiety supplement.

The herb *Centella asiatica* has been used traditionally as a mental tonic and there is evidence that Centella may improve the mental ability of children.

The herb Ashwagandha (*Withania somnifera*) has been used traditionally to reduce anxiety and stress and may be useful to support memory.

Valerian is a well-known herb that has been used traditionally for centuries for nervous debilities, failing reflexes, and as a natural sedative.

Omega-3 fatty acids from fish oils and certain vegetable oils are believed to improve brain function and decrease the risk of certain diseases.

Despite the protection guaranteed by the IDEA (Individuals With Disabilities Education Act) and Section 504 of the Rehabilitation Act of 1973, many children with ADD/ADHD continue to be denied access to an appropriate range of special education and/or related services. Myths and ignorance about ADD/ADHD continue, even though scientific research has documented ADD/ADHD as a neurological disability.

Instead of relying on the kindness of the government and your local school district, I suggest you begin treating your child's health conditions at home. Once you have discovered a proper overall treatment for your child, share it with others including your neighbors, your school, and your general community. For ADD/ADHD kids or adults, proper diet and nutrition is very important and critical for general health and the amelioration of debilitating symptoms.

Let's look more closely at some of the nutritional elements, including the vitamins, minerals, special nutrients, and herbal supplements that I recommend for ADD/ADHD conditions:

VITAMINS

VITAMIN A (RETINOL)

Importance: Necessary for growth and repair of body tissues; helps maintain smooth, soft, disease-free skin; helps protect the mucous membranes of the mouth, nose, throat and lungs, thereby reducing susceptibility to infections; protects against air pollutants; counteracts night-blindness and weak eyesight; aids in bone and teeth formation. Unlike large amounts or doses of vitamin A from fish-liver oil or synthetic sources, *beta carotene*, a form of vitamin A such as that contained in *Dunaliella Salina* or another pure, naturally occurring vegetable source, is non-toxic. Current medical research shows that foods rich in beta carotene will help reduce the risk of lung cancer and certain oral cancers.

Deficiency symptoms: Possible night blindness; increased susceptibility to infections; rough, dry, scaly skin; loss of smell and appetite; frequent fatigue; lack of tearing; defective teeth and gums, retarded growth. Any of these symptoms can contribute to the severity of ADD/ADHD symptoms and therefore vitamin A is important for the general health of ADD/ADHD kids and adults.

VITAMIN C (ASCORBIC ACID)

Importance: Essential for healthy teeth, gums and bones; helps heal wounds, scar tissue, and fractures; prevents scurvy; builds resistance to infection; aids in the prevention and treatment of the common cold; gives strength to blood vessels; aids in the absorption of iron. It is required for the synthesis of collagen, the intercellular "cement" which holds tissues together. It is also one of the major antioxidant nutrients. It prevents the conversion of nitrates (from tobacco smoke, smog, bacon, lunch meats and some vegetables) into cancer-causing substances. According to the late Dr. Linus Pauling, a prominent authority on vitamin C, vitamin C will decrease the risk of developing certain cancers by 75 percent. Vitamin C is known to reduce free radicals, which are toxic compounds that collect in the blood and body tissues due to stresses of all kinds, whether natural or induced by environmental and societal conditions. Vitamin C is important to help maintain health and can be used preventatively when additional stresses at work or school come into play or as a regular daily routine for those with ADD/ADHD conditions.

Deficiency symptoms: May lead to soft and bleeding gums, swollen or painful joints, slow-healing wounds and fractures, bruising, nosebleeds, tooth decay, loss of appetite, muscular weakness, skin hemorrhages, capillary weakness, anemia and impaired digestion.

VITAMIN E (TOCOPHEROL)

Importance: Vitamin E is a major anti-oxidant nutrient; retards cellular aging due to oxidation; supplies oxygen to the blood that is then carried to the heart and other organs, thus alleviating fatigue; aids in bringing nourishment to cells; strengthens the capillary walls and prevents the red blood cells from destructive poisons; prevents and dissolves blood clots; has also been used by doctors in helping prevent sterility, muscular dystrophy, calcium deposits in blood walls and heart conditions. For those with ADD/ADHD, vitamin E is another essential anti-stress vitamin and anti-oxidant that reduces fatigue and helps to eliminate free radical toxins from the body – both of which are vital to ameliorating ADD/ADHD symptoms.

Supplements can contain two forms of vitamin E – d-alpha-tocopherol and dl-alpha-tocopherol. What is the difference? Dl-alpha is synthetic and d-alpha is natural, usually from vegetable oils.

Deficiency symptoms: Lack of vitamin E may lead to a rupture of red blood cells, loss of reproductive powers, lack of sexual vitality, abnormal fat deposits in muscles, degenerative changes in the heart and other muscles; dry skin.

VITAMIN B_1 (THIAMINE)

Importance: Plays a key role in the body's metabolic cycle for generating energy; aids in the digestion of carbohydrates; essential for the normal functioning of the nervous system, muscles and heart; stabilizes the appetite; promotes growth and good muscle tone. Because vitamin B_1 is vital for proper nervous system functioning and growth, it must be included in a supplement program for those with ADD/ADHD.

Deficiency symptoms: Lack of B_1 may lead to loss of appetite; weakness and fatigue; paralysis and nervous irritability; insomnia; loss of weight; vague aches and pains; mental depression and constipation; heart and gastrointestinal problems.

VITAMIN B_2 (RIBOFLAVIN)

Importance: Necessary for carbohydrate, fat and protein metabolism; aids in the formation of antibodies and red blood cells; maintains cell respiration, necessary for the maintenance of good vision, skin, nails and hair; alleviates eye fatigue; promotes general health. All the B vitamins support each other and create a synergy for all of their functions. Like B_1, B_2

is vital for growth and should be included in dietary supplementation programs for everyone with ADD/ADHD.

Deficiency symptoms: Lack of vitamin B_2 may result in itching and burning eyes; cracks and sores in the mouth and lips; bloodshot eyes; purplish tongue; dermatitis; retarded growth; digestive disturbances; trembling; sluggishness; oily skin.

VITAMIN B_3 (NIACIN)

Importance: Improves circulation and reduces the cholesterol level in the blood; maintains the nervous system; helps metabolize protein, sugar and fat; reduces high blood pressure; increases energy through proper utilization of food; prevents pellagra; helps maintain a healthy skin, tongue and digestive system. B_3 is an essential vitamin for the nervous system. A healthy nervous system is vital for everyone, especially those with ADD/ADHD. A weak nervous system that is deficient in nutrients can contribute to ADD/ADHD symptoms, such as depression, rather than prevent them.

Deficiency symptoms: Lack of vitamin B_3 may result in pellagra, gastrointestinal disturbance, nervousness, headaches, fatigue, mental depression, vague aches and pains, irritability, loss of appetite, insomnia, skin disorders, muscular weakness, indigestion, bad breath, canker sores.

VITAMIN B_6 (PYRIDOXINE)

Importance: Necessary for the synthesis and breakdown of amino acids (the building blocks of protein); aids in fat and carbohydrate metabolism and the formation of antibodies;

maintains the central nervous system, aids in the removal of excess fluid in premenstrual women; promotes healthy skin; reduces muscle spasms, leg cramps, hand numbness, nausea and stiffness of hands; helps maintain a proper balance of sodium and phosphorus in the body. B_6 is vital for those with ADD/ADHD conditions because it is necessary for a healthy nervous system, and supports normal and calm behavior and routines.

Deficiency symptoms: Lack of vitamin B_6 may result in nervousness, insomnia, skin eruptions, loss of muscular control, anemia, mouth disorders, muscular weakness, dermatitis, arm and leg cramps, loss of hair, slow learning, and water retention.

VITAMIN B_{12} (CYANOCOBALAMIN)

Importance: Helps in the formation and regeneration of red blood cells, thus helping prevent anemia; necessary for carbohydrate, fat and protein metabolism; maintains a healthy nervous system; promotes growth in children; increases energy; needed for calcium absorption. For ADD/ADHD kids and adults, calcium supplementation is vital for growth and/or general health and specifically for the health of the brain and nervous system.

Deficiency symptoms: Lack of vitamin B_{12} may lead to pernicious anemia, poor appetite, growth failure in children, tiredness, brain damage, nervousness, neuritis, degeneration of spinal cord, depression, lack of balance.

VITAMIN B_5 (PANTOTHENIC ACID)

Importance: Participates in the release of energy from carbohydrates, fats and protein, aids in the utilization of vitamins; improves the body's resistance to stress; helps in cell building and the development of the central nervous system; helps the adrenal glands; fights infections by building antibodies. For those with ADD/ADHD conditions, this is an essential nutrient to prevent fatigue and to support a healthy nervous system.

Deficiency symptoms: Lack of vitamin B_5 may lead to painful and burning feet, skin abnormalities, retarded growth, dizzy spells, vomiting, digestive disturbances, restlessness, stomach stress, muscle cramps.

TRACE ELEMENTS ("MICROMINERALS")

ZINC

Importance: An antioxidant nutrient, necessary for protein synthesis; wound healing; vital for the development of the reproductive organs, prostate functions and male hormone activity; governs the contractility of muscles; important for blood stability; maintains the body's alkaline balance; helps in normal tissue function; aids in the digestion and metabolism of phosphorus. For those with ADD/ADHD conditions, zinc may help prevent a lack of alertness.

Deficiency symptoms: Lack of zinc may result in delayed sexual maturity, prolonged healing wounds, white spots on finger nails, retarded growth, stretch marks, fatigue, decreased alertness, susceptibility to infections.

COPPER

Importance: Necessary for the absorption and utilization of iron; helps oxidize vitamin C and works with vitamin C to form elastin, a chief component of the elastin muscle fibers throughout the body; aids in the formation of red blood cells; helps proper bone formation and maintenance. Copper is an important catalyst that helps other nutrients function properly.

Deficiency symptoms: Lack of copper may result in general weakness, impaired respiration, skin sores.

CHROMIUM

Importance: Works with insulin in the metabolism of sugar and stabilizes blood sugar levels; cleans the arteries by reducing cholesterol and triglyceride levels; helps transport amino acids to where the body needs them; helps control the appetite; medical research has shown that persons with low levels of chromium in their bodies are more susceptible to having cancer and heart problems and becoming diabetic. In ADD/ADHD conditions, chromium can help to balance blood sugar levels, reduce fatigue, and balance hunger cravings, which can help to calm and balance behaviors.

Deficiency symptoms: Lack of chromium may result in glucose intolerance in diabetics; arteriosclerosis, heart disease, depressed growth, obesity, tiredness.

OMEGA-3 FATTY ACIDS

Omega-3 fatty acids are polyunsaturated fats found in high concentrations in fish oils and certain vegetable oils such as flax seed, walnuts, and pumpkin seed.

Scientists are constantly discovering new health benefits for fish oils and certain vegetable oils and their essential fatty acids (EFAs, including omega-3s). In addition to their more notable properties as heart-healing substances, there is evidence that these fatty acids ease menstrual cramps and the pain and heavy bleeding of endometriosis. Omega-3s may even aid mental disorders such as schizophrenia; preliminary findings in studies of people with manic depression (bipolar disorder) link oil supplementation to fewer mood swings. Omega-3 fatty acids are essential as a nutritional approach to help improve the health of the brain and nervous system and reduce or help to prevent symptoms of ADD/ADHD.

AMINO ACIDS

Amino acids are vital for control of ADD/ADHD symptoms because they are essential for healthy brain and nervous-system function.

Proteins, vitamins, minerals, carbohydrates and fats are the essential nutrients that make up your body. They are responsible for growth and daily function. Proteins are essential components of muscle tissue, organs, enzymes, blood, antibodies, and neurotransmitters in the brain. Proteins are made from amino acids. Our bodies perform the process of creating proteins from the amino acids that we take in through food and supplementation. It is necessary, therefore, to constantly replace amino acids, especially the eight "essential" amino acids that the body cannot produce on its own, to nourish the body and repair and regenerate tissue. Although we obtain amino acids from food, especially fresh, whole organic food, proper dietary balance is rarely achieved. Much of the soil in which our food, even organic food, is grown today is significantly under-mineralized, and supplementation is important for keep the body in good health. Also, in times of physical and emotional stress, or in health conditions such as ADD/ADHD, the body requires more amino acids than can be obtained from food alone. Additionally, various health conditions and environmental factors, and a fast-paced lifestyle, may cause an imbalance of amino acids, which is challenging to good health and longevity.

Amino acids are the building blocks of the body. Besides building cells and repairing tissue, they form antibodies to combat invading bacteria and viruses; they are part of the enzyme and hormonal system; they build nucleoproteins (RNA and DNA); they carry oxygen throughout the body and participate in muscle activity. When protein is broken down by digestion, the result is 22 known amino acids. Eight are essential (cannot be manufactured by the body) and the rest are non-essential (can be manufactured by the body with proper nutrition).

KEY AMINO ACIDS FOR THE TREATMENT OF ADD/ADHD

L-CARNITINE

An amino acid which has been found to improve fat metabolism in the heart and other organs and tissues; reduces triglyceride and cholesterol levels, improves heart-muscle tolerance, prevents irregular heartbeat and angina, provides more energy for the heart and helps lower blood pressure.

TAURINE

A non-essential amino acid. Helps stabilize the excitability of membranes, which is extremely important in the control of epileptic seizures; aids in the clearing of free radical wastes. Taurine and sulfur are considered to be factors necessary for the control of many biochemical changes that take place in the aging process.

GAMMA AMINOBUTYRIC ACID (GABA)

GABA is a non-essential amino acid that functions as an inhibitory calming neurotransmitter in your brain. It is found in high concentrations only in your brain and eyes. It can be derived from protein foods or manufactured in your body from glutamic acid.

Its function is to decrease neuron activity and inhibit nerve cells from over-firing. Too much neuronal activity can lead to restlessness and insomnia, but GABA inhibits the number of nerve cells that fire in the brain and helps to induce sleep, uplift mood, and reduce anxiety.

GABA is usually deficient in both clinical and experimentally induced seizures. Low levels of GABA promote excitatory neurotransmitters. Low GABA levels have been found in the brains of patients with multiple sclerosis, action tremors, tardive dyskinesia, and other disorders of movement. Low GABA levels have been found in panic, anxiety, depression, alcoholism, and bipolar disorders.

GLYCINE

A non-essential amino acid. Helps trigger the release of oxygen creating energy required in the cell-making process; important in the manufacturing of hormones responsible for a strong immune system.

PHENYLALAINE

An essential amino acid. Used by the brain to produce norepinephrine, a chemical that transmits signals between nerve cells and the brain; keeps you awake and alert; reduces hunger pains, functions as an antidepressant and helps improve memory.

COENZYME Q10 (UBIQUINONE)

One of the world's most popular supplements, the chemical coenzyme Q10 has generated great excitement as a heart-disease remedy and a treatment for countless other conditions. The body naturally produces this compound, which has been dubbed "vitamin Q" because of its essential role in keeping all systems running smoothly. In fact, the scientists who identified coenzyme Q10 in 1957 initially honored its ubiquitous presence – it is found in every human cell and in all living organisms – by naming it "ubiquinone." A member of a family of compounds called quinines, coenzyme Q10 (sometimes called CoQ10) works in concert with enzymes (hence the name "coenzyme") to break down and convert food into energy. It is particularly abundant in high-energy-demanding cells, such as those found in the heart. In addition, coenzyme Q10 acts as a powerful antioxidant to prevent the cellular damage caused by unstable oxygen molecules called free radicals. For those with ADD/ADHD, Q10 is important for reducing the free radicals associated with "stress" conditions, preventing the associated toxicity and reducing overall chemical responses to stress, thereby supporting normal health and healthy behaviors.

HERBAL SUPPORT

Few people realize the value in herbs for treating ADD/ADHD. Still fewer understand what they are, how far back in history they have been used, from where they originate, or the extent to which herbs have influenced modern day medical practices.

First, what is an herb? Most modern definitions state that an herb is any part of the plant that is useful for healing, food, dye or colorants.

Herbalism is the practice and study of the uses of plants for the promotion of health.

Are herbs safe? The answer, in general, is yes – but they must be used with an understanding of their benefits. In all cases, if you are unsure whether an herb or any nutrient is useful or effective, consult your health professional before using it. Many herbs that are used today come from age-old traditions within medical systems dating back thousands of years, such as Oriental medicine. Traditional herbs, which have been used for various health conditions for centuries and have a history of safety, are the ones that I recommend for use in ADD/ADHD conditions. I prefer traditional herbs because doctors have used them in clinical practice for centuries, their effects are long known and they are not "new" or "experimental" in any way. I consider traditional herbs generally safe and efficacious if used correctly in properly compounded formulations designed by experts in the field of herbal medicine.

When confronted with a choice between the "synthetic" drug approach and the natural nutritional approach to ADD/ADHD conditions, I always prefer the natural approach. The natural approach, which can include herbal supplementation, is a much safer path than the non-natural, synthetic drug approach, which almost always leads to an accumulation of negative side effects and potentially serious health imbalances.

Here are the herbs I recommend for home use to help improve ADD/ADHD symptoms. Consult a qualified herbalist and/or doctor for the best and right dosages for your child.

BACOPA

Bacopa monnieria has been traditionally used to nourish the brain and to help support mental function, alertness, and memory.

In Oriental medical literature, Bacopa is known as Nir Brahmi, a reputed nervine tonic. B. monnieria L. has been widely used in the treatment of mental retardation, epilepsy and insanity in the traditional system of Indian medicine, and has been the focus of a 30-year study by the Central Drug Research Institute (CDRI) in India to establish the scientific basis of its action (more details in the Reference section, p. 117).

In another study, Bacopa was found to be effective in the revitalization of intellectual functions in children. The study concluded that the student children receiving Bacopa performed better on the testing and reaction timing.

A further study evaluated students with IQ testing after being given Bacopa (Brahmi) and it was concluded that IQ scores for the students who took Bacopa improved compared to the control group.

GOTU KOLA (CENTELLA ASIATICA)

This herb has been used traditionally for brain function including memory and stress.

Brain performance: John Heinerman, author of *Dr. Heinerman's Encyclopedia of Anti-Aging Remedies*, believes the "memory enhancing" attributes of Gotu kola may be attributed to the herb's ability to elevate blood sugar levels significantly. In addition, Gotu kola is very high in B-complex vitamins, which may help explain its positive effects on brain function. The B-complex vitamins help the body convert food into energy, and they are also responsible for nervous system function, both essential to a well-organized, clear-thinking brain. Gotu kola also contains triterpenoid compounds, which have a tranquilizing, anti-stress, and anti-anxiety effect while simultaneously stimulating mental function and all central nervous system functions.

In a clinical study, Gotu kola was observed to reduce hypertension.

Studies show that Gotu kola improves blood flow throughout the body, including the brain, by strengthening the veins and capillaries, and also promotes growth of connective tissues. Proponents believe Gotu kola's stimulating effect on circulation may help improve memory, and that by nourishing connective and fatty tissues in the brain, it enhances overall brain function, including memory.

ECLIPTA ALBA

Eclipta alba is used traditionally as a brain tonic and to support mental functioning.

ASHWAGANDA (WITHANIA SOMNIFERA)

Ashwagandha, *or Withania somnifera,* is used traditionally for support of mental functions and general strengthening.

Ashwagandha has traditionally been used to stabilize moods in patients with behavioral disturbances. Another study showed that Ashwagandha does indeed produce an anti-depressant and anti-anxiety effect comparable to the anti-depressant drug imipramine and the anti-anxiety drug lorazepam.

More details can be found in the Reference section on p. 117.

MUCUNA PRURIENS

Mucuna pruriens is a traditional herb used historically for various nervous-related conditions; it has been found to contain naturally occurring dopamine (L-Dopa and L-Dopa precursors or analogues). The lack of proper levels of L-Dopa in the brain is a sign of ADD/ADHD conditions.

How can we put natural dopamine back into our bodies? By supplementing our diets with natural botanicals that contain dopamine and dopamine precursors. In the body, dopamine converts to norepinephrine, as long as vitamin C is available, and finally to epinephrine. A norepinephrine deficiency can cause depression, a common symptom of ADD/ADHD. The original dopamine deficiency may be caused by a combination of factors: exposure to environmental pollutants, nutritional deficiencies, food or airborne allergies, the stress of a fast-paced lifestyle, gastrointestinal injury and genetic vulnerabilities. Combined, these may cause changes in brain chemistry, which can induce ADD/ADHD-related behavioral problems. More details can be found in the Reference section on p. 117.

AMLA FRUIT (EMBLICA OFFICINALIS)

Amla is considered to be one of the strongest traditional revitalizers, particularly for the blood, bones, liver and heart. It is an exceptionally rich source of naturally occurring vitamin C, containing 30 times the amount found in oranges. Amla is an excellent anti-oxidant and free-radical scavenger, significantly reducing the stress-related symptoms in ADD/ADHD patients.

Amla enhances production of red blood cells, strengthens the teeth, hair and nails, and regulates blood sugar. Recent scientific evidence shows that amla prevents lipid peroxidation, a condition that is a cause of atherosclerosis, which can lead to heart disease in cell membranes.

Scientists recently confirmed the potent anti-inflammatory action of amla in several animal studies. Researchers also recently confirmed the reputed cell- protective effects of this valuable herb, as well its demonstrably protective effects against melanoma.

HARITAKI (TERMINALIA CHEBULA)

Haritaki is a gentle laxative that nourishes the brain and nerves. In Asian medicine, Haritaki is called "the mother," and is thought to increase mental awareness.

NUTMEG (MYRISTICA FRAGRANS)

Nutmeg is first and foremost a pungent digestive aid. Asian

medicine uses nutmeg to promote the absorption of nutrients. It treats excess gas, and slows diarrhea.

It has also been used traditionally to quiet the mind and help prevent insomnia.

BIBITAKI (TERMINALIA BELERICA)

Bibitaki is a powerful rejuvenative herb that nourishes the body and promotes general health. Bibitaki has been shown in recent studies to protect the liver from damage.

CARDAMOM (ELETTARIA CARDAMOMUM)

Cardamom, a common spice used frequently in food preparation, is an excellent digestive enhancer, especially for cold and sweet food.

Cardamom is used in herbal medicine to treat gastralgia, enuresis (involuntary urination), spermatorrhea, phlegm, indigestion and gas.

Recent studies have shown that cardamom has pain-relieving, anti-inflammatory and antispasmodic effects.

For those interested in using the herbs and nutrients mentioned above for the supporting a relief of ADD/ADHD symptoms, there are supplements available that contain these ingredients available from your health professional, at natural food stores and through internet websites. More details can be found in the Reference section on p. 117 or by visiting www.papaschoice.com.)

8 Food Additives To Avoid

The following pages contain brief lists of ingredients that are often shown on food labels and should be avoided. (It is highly recommend that you start reading food and cosmetic product labels regularly, if you do not already do so, in order to avoid toxic and problem ingredients.)

Artificial Colorings

For many years, synthetic food dyes and artificial colorings have been suspected toxins or carcinogens (cancer-causing substances), and many have been banned. Many artificial food colors are used in American-made snacks, sodas, cakes, mixes and all kinds of junk foods. Artificial colors are mostly used in foods of questionable nutritional value; whenever possible, choose foods that contain none. Packaged foods purchased in health-food stores generally contain far fewer, if any, synthetic food dyes.

Some common names of artificial colors as found on labels:

Blue #1 (Erioglaucine)	
Blue #2 (Indigotine)	
Green #3 (Fast Green)	
Red # 3 (Erythrosin B)	
Yellow #6 (Sunset Yellow)	Banned in Norway.
Yellow #5 (Tartrazine)	Banned in Norway and Austria.
Red #40 (Allura Red)	Banned in Denmark, Belgium, France, Germany, Switzerland, Sweden, Austria and Norway.

The seven colorings listed above are the only artificial food colorings certified for consumption in the United States. Even so, they are all made from synthetic chemicals and I believe they should be avoided, especially by those with ADD/ADHD symptoms.

Cochineal, Carminic acid Carmines	
Red 2G	Banned in Australia.
Indigotine, Indigo carmine	Banned in Norway.
Brilliant blue FCF (FD&C Blue Dye No.1)	
Plain caramel	Dark brown color made from sucrose.
Titanium dioxide	White color used in toothpaste and white paint.
Iron oxides and hydroxides	

Other additives to avoid:

Aluminum salts	
Aspartame (marketed as Equal and NutraSweet) A	This sugar substitute should always be avoided as it is a proven carcinogen.
BHA and BHT	These two closely-related chemicals are added to oil-containing foods to prevent oxidation and retard rancidity. The International Agency for Research on Cancer, part of the World Health Organization, considers BHA to be possibly carcinogenic to humans, and the State of California has listed it as a carcinogen. Banned in Japan.

Caffeine	Especially to be avoided when "added" and not naturally occurring.
Monosodium Glutamate (MSG)	Also avoid hydrolyzed vegetable protein, or HVP, which may contain MSG.
Nitrite and nitrate	When nitrite combines with compounds called secondary amines, it forms nitrosamines, extremely powerful carcinogens.
Olestra	An artificial fat. Despite being approved as safe by the FDA, all snacks containing olestra must carry a warning label (similar to one found on cigarettes) that states: This Product Contains Olestra. Olestra may cause abdominal cramping and loose stools. Olestra inhibits the absorption of some vitamins and other nutrients. Vitamins A, D, E, and K have been added.
Potassium bromate	Banned virtually worldwide except in Japan and the United States. It is rarely used in California, because a cancer warning is required on the label.
Sulfites	A class of chemicals that can keep cut fruits and vegetables looking fresh.
Saccharin	Artificial sweetener.
Cyclamate	Artificial sweetener.
Acesulfame potassium, acesulfame K (marketed as Sunett and Sweet One)	Artificial sweetener.
Propyl gallate	Antioxidant.

Food Additives That Have Been Banned

The food and chemical corporations have for many years told us, not surprisingly, that food additives are tested and safe.

But the history of food additives includes many that were found to be very toxic and to pose severe health risks such as cancer. Those listed below have been banned. Always question safety claims made by companies with commercial interests who have only their own bottom line as a priority. Food additives may help bring them profit, but they may also be harmful to your health and health of your children.

Agene (nitrogen trichloride)	Flour bleaching and aging agent
Artificial colorings	Butter yellow
	Green #1
	Orange #1
	Orange #2
	Orange B
	Red #1
	Red #2
	Red #4
	Red #32
	Sudan #1
	Violet #1
	Yellow #1
	Yellow #2
	Yellow #3
	Yellow #4
Cinnamyl anthranilate	Flavoring and fragrance agent
Cobalt salts	Stabilizer for beer foam
Diethyl pyrocarbonate (DEPC)	Preservative
Dulcin (p-ethoxy-phenylurea)	Artificial sweetener
Ethylene glycol	Solvent humectant
Monochloroacetic acid	Preservative
Polyoxyethylene-8-stearate	Emulsifier
Safrole	Flavoring agent

TOXIC INGREDIENTS IN SOAPS, SHAMPOOS AND OTHER PERSONAL CARE PRODUCTS

Here are some synthetic, toxic ingredients found commonly in *cosmetics, soaps, shampoos and personal care products* that should be avoided (read the product labels!).

- Methyl, propyl, butyl and ethyl parabens
- Sodium lauryl sulfate (SLS, also known as sodium laurel sulfate) and sodium laureth sulfate (SLES, also know as sodium lauryl esther sulfate)
- Propylene glycol (PG), polyethylene glycol (PEG), butylene glycol (BG), and thylene Glycol (EG): PG, PEG, BG and EG are all petroleum derivatives that act as solvents, surfactants, and wetting agents
- Petrolatum and mineral oil: Mineral oil is a derivative of crude oil and petrolatum is mineral-oil jelly. Both are used industrially as lubricants. Products that contain mineral oil and petrolatum often create the very conditions they are intended to treat
- Imidazolidinyl urea and diazolidinyl urea
- DEA (diethanolamine), MEA (monoethanolamine) and TEA (triethanolamine): Some other names: cocamide DEA or MEA, DEA-cetyl phosphate, DEA oleth-3 phosphate, myristamide DEA, stearamide MEA, lauramide DEA, linoleamide MEA, oleamide DEA, TEA-lauryl Sulfate
- Butylated hydroxianisole (BHA) and butylated hydroxy-toluene (BHT): BHA and BHT 8
- Phthalates
- Synthetic colors (see page 95)

9
Conclusion

I was moved to write this book by my anger at our nation's growing tendency to use harmful prescription drugs as a first course of action in the treatment of disease. This is an appalling, completely inappropriate solution for what I see as basic problems in the way we are living today. The truth, confirmed by nearly every parent I speak with, is that what parents *really* want are easy solutions – not easy and harmful ones. But harmful disguised as easy is what you are getting when you use pharmaceuticals to address children with ADD/ADHD.

Not only are these substances controlling and addictive, but they have both known and unknown deleterious affects. With each prescription we are taking an innocent, vulnerable child and running a serious risk of creating a zombie-like child with a high likelihood of leading a drug-dependent life. This is not health, nor is it a permanent solution.

It's up to us as parents to seek proper and appropriate solutions rather than risk significantly compromising our child's life, creativity, and ability to function as a healthy adult. We need to ask questions rather than simply accept what is told to us. If your first instinct was "No!" when the doctor suggested pharmaceuticals, then follow it. Trust me, once you make the basic but critical decision to find alternative, healthy ways to address your child's illness, things become easier.

Do your research and talk to several qualified medical professionals who support your intuition that drugs are not the right and best solution for you and your child. I'm here to make it easy on you. Visit my website, www.papaschoice.com, for valuable information in determining your next steps. Purchase my recipe book so that you have access to easy and healthy meals in minutes. Read other books that present good, commonsense information, and then formulate your own opinions. Lastly, consider forming groups with other parents who also wish to resolve the ADD/ADHD challenge without the use of drugs. Get the support that you need; you will be grateful that you did.

Lastly, I encourage you to exhaust every option that you have prior to subscribing to a drug protocol. Children first need healthy and balanced diets with supplementation, plenty of outdoor time including time for rest and relaxation, and a loving and nurturing environment that minimizes stress levels. Together, we can create a happy, drug-free existence for our children.

The choices are ours to take. We can turn our backs on "chemical parenting" and the use of drugs to address ADD/ADHD, or we can raise our children free from ADD/ADHD symptoms by applying the natural approaches discussed in this book. Even if drugs become necessary as an emergency measure, we can eventually free ourselves from drug dependency by implementing and reinforcing commonsense approaches – wholesome food choices, supplementation, toxin-free environments and healthy living.

Taking the natural path is actually less costly (from many viewpoints), easier and more beneficial. Our entire society, and the environment, will benefit from our natural and healthy choices. Most importantly, you and your family will reap many rewards by choosing to eliminate ADD/ADHD symptoms naturally – the net result being a great improvement in the quality of your life.

It is my sincere wish that you and your family and everyone in your circle of influence benefit from the recommendations in this book. May you and your children experience the joy of focused health and happiness always.

Yours in health,

Dr. Michael Papa

10
RECIPES

Preparing healthy meals can be challenging in our fast-paced, busy world. Below are some quick, easy and healthy recipes that will help you and your family on the road to wellness. The more that you can do to ensure a balanced diet full of nutrient-rich fruits, vegetables and grains, the better you will feel. Enjoy!

Logon to my website www.papaschoice.com to order a copy of my recipe book, *Delicious and Healthy Recipes for People Living with ADD/ADHD.*

SESAME POTATOES

4 baking potatoes
2 tablespoons of good oil (Olive oil or sunflower oil)
2 tablespoons sesame seeds
1 cup cheese

Directions:

1. Pre-heat oven to 400°F
2. Scrub the potatoes and cut parallel slices. Brush with oil and roll firmly into the sesame seeds.
3. Bake for about 1 hour, until tender inside and crispy brown outside.
4. Cut small slices of cheese to fit inside the opened-out potato slices. Return to the oven for a few minutes until the cheese melts. Serve hot.

BANANA AND LEMON DRINK

2 large bananas
3 teaspoons lemon juice
2 tablespoons raw honey

Directions:

1. Blend all the ingredients together until frothy.
2. Serve with slices of whole grain toast.

STIR FRY VEGETABLES

1 pound (16 oz.) mixed vegetables
3 tablespoons good oil
1 pinch sea salt
1 teaspoon raw cane sugar
1 tablespoon natural soy sauce
2 pinches ground ginger
3 teaspoons arrowroot (flour)
Water as needed

Directions:

1. Mix your own vegetables, such as bean sprouts, spring onions (scallions), celery, broccoli, cauliflower, carrots, turnips, mushrooms or cabbage. Cut them into very thin slices, or small diagonal chunks.
2. Heat the oil in a pan or wok then add the 'hard' vegetables first and fry at a high heat for a minute, then add the soft vegetables and fry for 2 minutes.
3. Add the salt, sugar, soy sauce, ginger and arrowroot mixture. Mix well and cook until the sauce thickens. Serve hot with organic brown rice.

VEGE-BURGERS

12 ounces (1½ cups) of Meat Substitute, vegetable source loose burger
1 small onion, finely chopped or minced
1 tablespoon chopped parsley
1 tablespoon of whole grain flour to bind
3 tablespoons olive oil
Sea salt and freshly ground pepper to taste

Directions:

1. Mix together all the ingredients except the oil.
2. Shape into four rounds. Dust with flour if necessary.
3. Heat the oil in a frying pan and cook the burgers for approximately 8 minutes each side, or until cooked through. (Reduce the heat if they are browning too quickly.)
4. Serve with whole grain buns with tomato, lettuce, and natural source condiments such as organic ketchup and mustard.

RICE SALAD

1 pound (16 oz.) brown rice
2 scallions finely chopped
1 small clove garlic, crushed
2 sticks celery, finely chopped
1 carrot, finely chopped
6 black olives, stoned
3 tablespoon olive oil
1 tablespoon lemon juice
1 teaspoon basil
Sea salt and freshly ground pepper

Directions:

1. Boil the rice until tender, but still firm.
2. While the rice is still warm add the remaining ingredients and season to taste.

CARROT AND LEMON SOUP

1 pound (16 oz.) prepared vegetables (e.g. 1 pound: 1 onion, 2 stalks of celery and 6 medium-sized carrots)
3 tablespoons virgin olive oil or butter
2 teaspoons grated lemon rind
1 tablespoon lemon juice
1 bay leaf
3 cups filtered water
Sea salt and freshly ground pepper to taste

Directions:

1. Chop onion, celery and carrots finely and sauté gently in oil until the vegetables begin to soften, about 5-10 minutes.
2. Add half of the grated lemon rind, the bay leaf and water, and simmer for about 20 minutes, until cooked.
3. Blend, then add the rest of the lemon rind, and the lemon juice and seasoning to taste.
4. Serve sprinkled with chopped parsley. Will freeze.

BEAN SALAD

1 pound (16 oz.) cooked beans (kidney beans or a mixture of red, white and green beans)
2 tablespoons olive oil
1 teaspoon lemon juice
1 tablespoon chopped parsley
1 clove garlic (optional)
Sea salt and freshly ground pepper to taste

Directions:

1. Mix all the other ingredients well together while the beans are still warm. Chill in the refrigerator before serving.

PASTA SALAD

2 cups pasta whole grain pasta shapes (such as butterfly or other)
2 cups chopped broccoli chunks
2 carrots, grated
1 cup (7 oz.) of pineapple chunks in own juice
1 cup bean sprouts
1 tablespoon natural soy sauce (without preservatives)
6 tablespoon organic sunflower or other good oil (Olive, flax or sunflower oil)

Directions:

1. Cook the whole grain pasta according to directions on the package. Drain well and set aside.
2. Cook the broccoli chunks in boiling water for about 3 minutes, then drain and set aside.
3. In a large bowl, mix the pasta, carrots, pineapple and bean sprouts and dressing ingredients together.
4. Add to the cooked pasta with the broccoli. Toss to Coat. Cool and serve.

NATURAL MARZIPAN TREATS

1 cup (4 oz.) Almonds
1/3 cup (3 oz.) raw honey

Directions:

1. Grind the whole or pieces of almonds into a fine powder using a coffee grinder or blender.
2. Put the almond flour into a bowel and add the honey working it into a paste. You can do this with other nuts, as well.
3. Makes a special treat and is great on whole grain toast as a natural snack.

ALPINE BREAKFAST CEREAL

½ cup unsweetened granola of your choice
1 grapefruit, peeled and segmented
1 pear, peeled and chopped
2 tablespoons (30g/10 oz.) chopped dates or figs
3 tablespoons (30g/10 oz.) nuts of choice (walnuts)
Honey to taste
Yogurt

Directions:

1. Place granola in a bowl.
2. Add the chopped pear to prevent it discoloring.
3. Gently mix the rest of the ingredients with the granola and honey
4. If possible, leave in the refrigerator or in a cool place for an hour before serving, or keep overnight in the refrigerator so that it will be ready for breakfast.

LEMON SHORTBREAD

½ cup (4 oz.) butter
⅓ cup (3 oz.) raw cane sugar or fructose
2 teaspoons lemon juice and grated rind of lemon
1 cup (4 oz.) whole grain flour
½ cup (2 oz.) rice flour

Directions:

1. Cream together softened butter and sugar.
2. Add juice and rind of lemon, then the whole grain flour and rice flour.
3. Rub the mixture together with your fingers until it forms a shortbread dough. Roll it out and cut into fingers. Place into a greased baking pan and bake for 10-12 minutes at 325°F. Cool and store in an airtight container.

HUMMUS

1/2 cup (4oz.) dried chick peas (garbanzo beans), OR
1 – 8 oz. can of organic garbanzo beans
1 clove garlic
2 tablespoons olive oil
1 tablespoon sesame paste (Tahini)
Juice of a large lemon
1/2 teaspoon Sea salt (or to taste)
1 tablespoon chopped parsley

Directions:

1. Soak the chick peas (garbanzos) overnight. Drain, cover with fresh water, and bring to a boil.
2. Simmer until tender, 1-2 hours depending on the batch, or cook in a pressure cooker for 30 minutes. Set aside.
3. Place the garlic, oil, sesame paste and lemon juice into the blender. Blend together then gradually add the chick peas, adding some of the cooking liquid to enable the blender to work.
4. Add Sea salt and more lemon juice to taste if necessary. Sprinkle chopped parsley on top.

APPENDIXES

A. A REVIEW OF MEDICATIONS

This section is devoted to a review of common ADD/ADHD drug medications, their dosages, effects and side effects (secondary or unwanted effects).

Methylphenidate (Ritalin, Methylin)

Form: Short-acting tablets administered by mouth. Methylphenidate: 5mg, 10mg and 20mg.

Dosage: Varies by individual. Usually between 2.5-20mg per dose. Effective dose does not necessarily correlate with age, body weight or severity of ADD/ADHD symptoms. Usually the physician prescribes a small starting dose and then gradually increases it to find the most effective dose that will not produce excessive adverse effects.

Duration of action: Rapid-acting methylphenidate starts to work in 15-20 minutes and lasts about 3.5-4 hours. Because of its relatively short action, this form of methylphenidate wears off at night and is started again when taken in the morning. Research suggests that short-acting methylphenidate works best for most persons when taken three times daily.

Possible side effects: Moderate appetite suppression, mild sleep disturbances, transient weight loss and irritability. "Rebound effect" can occur – anger, frustration or sadness –

for a period of about one hour when the effect of medication wears off. When the dosage is too high, motor tics may be unmasked, or agitation, depression or lethargy may occur until the dose wears off. These are usually managed by lowering the dose. Tics will usually disappear if the dose is lowered.

Contraindications: Anxiety, tension, agitation, thyrotoxicosis, tachyarrhythmias, severe angina pectoris and glaucoma. Hypersensitivity to methylphenidate. Also contraindicated in patients with motor tics or with a family history or diagnosis of Tourette's syndrome.

Extended-Delivery Forms Of Methylphenidate

To avoid the need for taking short-acting methylphenidate 3-4 times daily, several new long-acting delivery systems have been developed. Each of the systems described below delivers the same medicine used in short-acting methylphenidate tablets, but does so in a way designed to give extended coverage so a child can get through a school day without having to take pills at school.

Concerta, a new osmotic release system for methylphenidate approved by the FDA in September 2000. This capsule contains three chambers, two filled with different concentrations of methylphenidate and one with a polymer substance that expands when a liquid comes in contact with it. An initial dose of methylphenidate is released from the outer coating soon after the capsule is ingested. As the polymer substance expands in response to liquids absorbed from the digestive tract, it gradually pushes the medication in the two internal chambers out of the capsule, like a piston, through a laser-drilled hole in one end of the capsule. Concerta delivers methylphenidate in an ascending profile. This means that an 18mg caplet provides 4mg methylphenidate initially and delivers the rest of the methylphenidate over the course of the day. An 18mg caplet of Concerta is equivalent to 5mg of Ritalin given three times per day. Concerta is designed to be effective for about 10-12 hours from ingestion, but individual results may vary. Concerta capsules should not be opened or chewed.

Form: 18mg, 27mg, 36mg and 54mg capsules. (Each 18mg is equivalent to about 5mg of short-acting methylphenidate given three times a day.)

Metadate-CD, an extended-delivery capsule approved by the FDA in April 2001, contains many tiny beads containing methylphenidate. Beads have various types of coatings so they can release 30 percent of the methylphenidate dose immediately and then continue to release methylphenidate over an extended period of time designed to cover a school day. Typically, Metadate-CD provides about eight hours of coverage. These capsules should not be chewed, but they may be opened and sprinkled at the direction of a physician.

Form: 20 mg CD capsule

Ritalin LA is another extended-delivery capsule form of methylphenidate. It also consists of two types of tiny beads in a capsule, but is unique in that the amount of methylphenidate released immediately is the same amount released four hours after the dose. Therefore, Ritalin LA delivers 50 percent of its methylphenidate initially and 50 percent approximately four hours later. This delivery system mimics Ritalin given twice a day, thus giving approximately eight hours worth of coverage.

Form: 20mg, 30mg and 40mg capsules.

Methylphenidate SR 20 (methylphenidate sustained release) and Ritalin SR 20, the earliest form of extended release methylphenidate, uses a wax matrix to deliver two doses from one pill. An SR 20 tablet releases about 10mg of methylphenidate within about one hour after ingestion and then releases another 10 mg between three and four hours later. It is intended to last six to eight hours. Clinicians report that this preparation works well for some individuals, but is unsatisfactory for many others because it may release too quickly or unevenly. The dosage is individualized. Possible side effects are the same as methylphenidate.

Form: 20mg tablets.

Metadate ER, Methylin ER: similar to the Ritalin SR tablet.

Form: 10mg and 20mg tablets.

AMPHETAMINE & AMPHETAMINE DERIVATIVES

Adderall (Mixed salts of a single-entity amphetamine product)

Form: Double-scored tablets administered by mouth: 5mg, 7.5mg, 10mg, 12.5mg, 15mg, 20mg and 30mg.

Dosage: Varies by individual.

Duration of action: Variable. Depending on dose, may last between three and a half to eight hours.

Possible side effects: Increased heart rate, insomnia, anorexia (loss of appetite), vertigo, headache, diarrhea, sweating, sexual dysfunction, dry mouth, irritability, tremor, euphoria. Less common: stomach upsets, nervousness, dilated pupils, teeth-grinding, urinary retention, pyrexia, tachycardia, tics, urticaria, increased urination (perhaps due to increased amounts of water ingestion), emotional numbness, detachment from reality.

Contraindications: Adderall (and any other amphetamine) must not be taken within one or two weeks of taking an antidepressant of the monoamine oxidase inhibitor (MAOI) class. Otherwise a very serious condition known as "serotonin syndrome" can result.

Adderall XR, extended release capsule approved by the FDA for ADD/ADHD in 2001. Mixed salts of amphetamine used are contained in tiny beads within a capsule. About half of the beads release within an hour; the rest release about three and a half hours later to provide coverage for approximately 10 hours.

Form: Capsules administered by mouth: 5mg, 10mg, 15mg, 20mg, 25mg and 30mg.

Duration of action: 10-12 hours.

Dextroamphetamine (Dexedrine, Dextrostat)

Form: Short-acting tablets administered by mouth: 5mg and 10mg tablets.

Dosage: Varies by individual. Average: 2.5-10mg.

Duration of action: Rapid onset of action, 20-30 minutes. Lasts about four to five hours.

Possible side effects: Same as methylphenidate.

Dextroamphetamine spansules (Dexedrine), sustained release capsules. Each spansule releases about half its face value dose in about one hour and then releases the balance about three and a half hours later. Thus a 5mg spansule actually releases 2.5mg initially and 2.5mg later. It does not provide the equivalent of 5g throughout the duration of its action.

Form: Long-acting, administered by mouth.
Dextroamphetamine spansules: 5mg, 10mg and 15mg.

Dosage: Varies by individual. Average: 5-20mg.

Duration of action: Varies by individual. Usually lasts six to eight hours but individual reaction may vary from several hours to the whole day.

Possible side effects: Similar to those of methylphenidate.

Pemoline (Cylert)

Pemoline has been used for the management of ADD/ADHD symptoms, but it has the potential for causing serious liver damage. FDA approval for pemoline was withdrawn in 2005 in response to pressure from public advocacy groups

SELECTIVE NOREPINEPHRINE REUPTAKE INHIBITORS

Atomoxetine (Strattera)

Approved by the FDA for the treatment of ADD/ADHD in November 2002. Atomoxetine acts as a highly specific reuptake inhibitor for norepinephrine and seems to have little effect on other neurotransmitters.

Form: Capsules administered by mouth: 10mg, 18mg, 25mg, 40mg and 60mg.

Dosage: The recommended initial dose is 0.5mg/kg/day, increasing to find the minimum effective dose up to a maximum of 1.2mg/kg/day.

Duration of action: Most patients appear to achieve 24-hour coverage from dosing one or two times a day.

Effect: Lower doses may improve ADD/ADHD symptoms within several days, but may take one to three weeks for full effect. Higher doses may improve depressive symptoms and mood swings.

Possible side effects: Nervousness, sleep problems, fatigue, stomach upset, dizziness and dry mouth.

Nortriptyline (various brands), imipramine (Tofranil), desipramine (Norpramin)

Form: Tablets administered by mouth: 10mg, 25mg, 50mg and 100mg.

Dosage: Varies by individual.

Duration of action: Variable. Often has 24-hour effect.

Effect: Lower doses may improve ADD/ADHD symptoms within several days, but may take one to three weeks for full effect. Higher doses may improve depressive symptoms and mood swings.

Possible side effects: Nervousness, sleep problems, fatigue, stomach upset, dizziness, dry mouth and accelerated heart rate. May affect conduction time of the heart, leading to irregular heart rate. In rare cases, may affect blood count. Should not be abruptly discontinued. Desipramine has been associated with deaths from cardiac problems. Most physicians do not use this medication with prepubescent children.

OTHER ANTIDEPRESSANTS

Bupropion (Wellbutrin)

Approved by the FDA for the treatment of depression in adults and for nicotine cessation treatment. It is not approved for ADD/ADHD.

Form: 75mg and 100mg tablets. 100mg and 150mg extended release.

Dosage: Varies by individual.

Duration of action: About four to six hours in short-acting form; six to eight hours in long-acting form.

Effect: Improves symptoms of ADD/ADHD and can affect depressive moods.

Possible side effects: Difficulty sleeping and headache.

Clonidine (Catapres)

Form: Clonidine is available in patches applied to back of shoulder or tablets administered by mouth: 0.1mg, 0.2mg and 0.3mg.

Dosage: Varies by individual. The Clonidine patch is available in three strengths.

Duration of action: Patches last five or six days. Tablets last four to six hours.

Effect: Often will improve excessive hyperactivity or insomnia associated with ADD/ADHD, but has demonstrated effectiveness for improving inattention symptoms. May decrease facial and vocal tics in Tourette's syndrome. Often has positive side effect on oppositional defiant behavior and may be beneficial for management of excessive anger.

Possible side effects: Major side effect is fatigue, though this will usually disappear over time. Other side effects may include dizziness, dry mouth, increased activity, irritability or behavior problems. Overdose may cause excessive sedation or other serious problems. Should not be stopped suddenly. Physician should be consulted prior to discontinuation of medication to prevent "rebound hypertension" or other effects.

Guanfacine (Tenex)

Form: 1mg tablets taken by mouth.

Dosage: Varies by individual.

Duration of action: six to eight hours.

Effect: Often will improve excessive hyperactivity or insomnia associated with ADD/ADHD, but has demonstrated effectiveness for improving inattention symptoms. May decrease facial and vocal tics in Tourette's syndrome. Often has positive side effects on oppositional defiant behavior and may be beneficial for management of excessive anger.

Possible side effects: Major side effect is fatigue, though this will usually disappear over time. Other side effects may include dizziness, dry mouth, increased activity, irritability or behavior problems. Physician should be consulted prior to discontinuation of medication to prevent "rebound hypertension" or other effects.

B. RESOURCES

DR. MICHAEL PAPA'S WEBSITE: www.papaschoice.com
Further information on Dr. Papa's approach, including an online questionnaire and information on nutritional supplements.

GENERAL INFORMATION ABOUT ADD/ADHD
http://www.loc.gov/rr/scitech/tracer-bullets/adhdtb.html#addinfo
The above site provides a list of organizations to contact.

GENERAL HEALTH
American Heart Association: http://www.americanheart.org/
American Cancer Association: http://www.cancer.org

BOOKS

Peter R. Breggin & Dick Scruggs. *Talking Back to Ritalin: What Doctors Aren't Telling You About Stimulants and ADHD.* Perseus Publishing, Cambridge, MA. 2001.

Doris Rapp. *Is this your Child?* Quill (Harper Paperbacks), New York, NY. 1991.

Doris Rapp. *Our Toxic World: A Wake-Up Call.* Environmental Research Foundation, Buffalo, NY. 2003.

Randall Fitzgerald. *The Hundred-Year Lie: How Food and Medicine Are Destroying Your Health.* Dutton Adult. 2006.

Michael F. Jacobson, Ph.D. and Bruce Maxwell. *What Are We Feeding our Kids?* Workman Publishing Company, New York, NY. 1994.

Rachel F. Heller, M.D. and Richard Heller, M.D. *Carbohydrate Addicted Kids: Help Your Child or Teen Break Free of Junk Food and Sugar Cravings – for Life!* Harper Paperbacks, New York, NY. 1998.

PARENTING RESOURCES

The STEP program (Systematic Training for Effective Parenting): http://www.ciccparenting.org/StepPrograms.aspx

FURTHER INFORMATION ON RITALIN

http://www.drugabuse.gov/Infofacts/Ritalin.html
http://www.rxlist.com/cgi/generic/methphen.htm
http://www.mentalhealth.com/drug/p30-r03.html
The above sites can provide information on other drugs used in treating ADD/ADHD.

FOOD COLORINGS AND HYPERACTIVITY

http://www.chem-tox.com/pregnancy/artificial.htm
http://www.diet-studies.com/adhd.html

CHILDHOOD OBESITY

http://www.cdc.gov/HealthyYouth/overweight/index.htm

CAMPAIGN TO BAN JUNK FOOD IN UK SCHOOLS

http://www.spiegel.de/international/1,1518,348368,00.html
http://news.bbc.co.uk/1/hi/education/4995268.stm

WILLIAM J. CLINTON FOUNDATION

http://www.clintonfoundation.org/cf-pgm-hs-hk-home.htm

C. REFERENCES

Further information and technical references related to recommended nutritional supplements

AMINO ACIDS

Bornstein, R. et al, *Plazma Amino Acids in Attention Deficit Disorder,* Psychiatry Research, 1990 33(3), 301-306.

McConnell, H., *Catecholamine Metabolism in the Attention Deficit Disorder: Implications for the use of Amino Acid Precursor Therapy,* Medical Hypotheses, 1985 17(4), 305-311.

Nemzer, E. et al, *Amino Acid Supplementation as Therapy for Attention Deficit Disorder,* Journal of American Academy of Child and Adolescent Psychiatry, 1986 25(4), 509-513.

HERBS

Bacopa

Scientists at the Central Drug and Research institute (CDRI) in India have isolated and characterized the two major compounds of Bacopa monnieria: Baccoside A and Baccoside B. The first schedule of clinical trials induced a labile behavior using a shock-motivated brightness-discrimination reaction. The Bacopa-treated group showed a better acquisition, improved retention and delayed extinction ($p < 0.01$-0.05). Similarly, in an active conditioned flight reaction, the Bacopa-treated subjects showed a shorter reaction time than the controls ($p < 0.01$). Also, in the continuous avoidance response the Bacopa-treated group performed better than the controls ($p < 0.01 - 0.05$).

Sharma, R., *"Efficacy of Bacopa monnieri in Revitalizing Intellectual Functions in Children,* Indian Journal Medical Research, Jan-June, 1987.

Abhang, R. *"Study of Evaluate the effect of a Micro...Medicine Derived from Brahmi...on the Students of Average Intelligence"*, JRAS, Vol. 14, No. 102, pp. 10-24, 1992.

Gotu kola

Belcaro, G., *"Efficacy of Centellase in the Treatment of Venous Hypertension Evaluated,"* Current Therapeutic Research, Vol. 46, No. 6, December 1989.

Cesarone, M.R., et al. *"The microcirculatory activity of Centella asiatica in venous insufficiency. A double-blind study,"* Minerva Cardioangiol, June 1994, 42(6):299-304.

Ashwagandha (Withania somnifera)

Researchers at Banaras Hindu University in Varanasi, India, and from the Drug Research and Development Center in Calcutta, India, discovered that some of the chemicals in Ashwagandha are powerful antioxidants. They tested these compounds on rats for their positive effects on brain function and found an increase in three natural antioxidants – superoxide dismutase, catalase and glutathione peroxidase. According to the researchers, "These findings are consistent with the therapeutic use of *Withania somnifera* (Ashwagandha) as a rejuvenator in Ayurvedic (Indian traditional) medicine. The antioxidant effect of active principles of W. somnifera may explain, at least in part, the reported anti-stress, cognition-facilitating, anti-inflammatory and anti-aging effects produced by them in experimental animals, and in clinical situations."

Another study examined Ashwagandha's effect on copper-induced lipid peroxidation and antioxidant enzymes in aging spinal cords of laboratory mice. The herb produced a strong antioxidant effect and stopped the lipid peroxidation, which, in humans, is a cause of atherosclerosis leading to heart disease.

Researchers from the University of Leipzig in Germany wanted to find out which neurotransmitters were influenced by Ashwagandha. After injecting some of the compounds found in Ashwagandha into rats, they examined slices of the animals' brains and found an increase in acetylcholine receptor activity. Acetylcholine is the most abundant and essential neurotransmitter in the brain that is responsible for numerous functions, including many related to cognition and memory. It is released into the synapse, or space between two nerve cells, where it stimulates the transfer of nerve impulses from one nerve cell to another. According to the researchers, the increase in acetylcholine receptor capacity might partly explain the cognition-enhancing and memory-improving effects of extracts from Ashwagandha observed in animals and humans.

Singh, B., Chandan, B.K., Gupta, D.K., Adaptogenic activity of a novel with anolide-free aqueous fraction from the roots of Withania somnifera Dun. (Part II). Phytotherapy Research, May 2003, 17(5), 531-6.

Bhattacharya, S.K., Muruganandam, A.V., Adaptogenic activity of Withania somnifera: an experimental study using a rat model of chronic stress. Pharmacology Biochemistry & Behavior, June 2003, 75(3), 547-55.

Mehta, A.K., Binkley, P., Gandhi, S.S., Ticku, M.K., Pharmacological effects of Withania somnifera root extract on GABAA receptor complex, Indian Journal Medical Research, August 1991, 94:312-5.

Bhattacharya, S.K., Bhattacharya, A., Sairam, K., Ghosal, S., Anxiolytic-antidepressant activity of Withania somnifera glycowithanolides: an experimental study. Phytomedicine, December 2000, 7(6):463-9.

Bhattacharya, S., Goel, R., Kaur, R., Ghosal, S., Anti-stress Activity of Sitoindosides VII and VIII, New Acylsterylglucosides from Withania Somnifera. Phytotherapy Research, 1987, 1:32-39.

Bhattacharya, A., Ghosal, S., Bhattacharya, S.K., Anti-oxidant effect of Withania somnifera glycowithanolides in chronic footshock stress-induced perturbations of oxidative-free radical scavenging enzymes and lipid peroxidation in rat frontal cortex and striatum. Journal Ethnopharmacology, January 2001, 74(1):1-6.

Schliebs, R., Liebmann, A., Bhattacharya, S.K., Kumar, A., Ghosal, S., Bigl, V., Systemic administration of defined extracts from Withania somnifera (Indian Ginseng) and Shilajit differentially affects cholinergic but not glutamatergic and GABAergic markers in rat brain. Neurochem International, February 1997, 30(2):181-90.

Kuboyama, T., Tohda, C., Zhao, J., Nakamura, N., Hattori, M., Komatsu, K., Axon- or dendrite-predominant outgrowth induced by constituents from Ashwagandha. Neuroreport, October 7, 2002, 13(14):1715-20.

Mucuna pruriens and L-Dopa:

Mahajani, S., Doshl, V., *Bioavailability of L-dopa from HP 200. Seed Powder of Mucuna pruriens...a Phramacokinetic and Pahmacodynamic Study*, Dept. of Neurol. S. Illinois Univ., Phytotherapy Research, Vol. 10, 254-256, 1996.

Manyan, B., *Mucuna pruriens Proves More Effective than (synthetic) L-dopa in Parkinson's Disease,* Dept. Neur., S. Illinois Univ., Phytotherapy Research, Vol. 11, 419-423, 1997.

Amla fruit

Bhattacharya, A., Chatterjee, A., Ghosal, S., Bhattacharya, S.K., Antioxidant activity of active tannoid principles of Emblica officinalis (amla). Indian Journal Experimental Biology, July 1999, 37(7):676-80.

Biswas, S., Talukder, G., Sharma, A., Protection against cytotoxic effects of arsenic by dietary supplementation with crude extract of Emblica officinalis fruit. Phytotherapy Research, September 1999, 13(6):513-6.

ADDITIONAL REFERENCES

Rimeau L., Allopathic Special Edition Review: ADD Protocol, Journal Botanical Medicine, Vol. 2, 24-28, 1996.

Kirschmann, G.J., *Nutrition Almanac*, McGraw-Hill, 1996.

Alakananda, D., Journal Botanical Medicine, Vol. 2, No.1, 1994.

Abhang, R., Study to Evaluate the effect of...Brahmi (Bacopa monnieri) on Students of Average Intelligence, JRAS, Vol. 14, Pgs. 10-24, 1992.

Sharma, R., Chaturvedi, C., Inst. Med. Science, BHU, Varanasi, Efficacy of Bacopa monnieri for Revitalizing Intellectual Functions in Children, Journ. Edu. Ind. Med., Jan-Jun, 1987.

Singh, R., Inst. Med. Science, BHU, Varanasi, Anti-Anxiety effect of...Brahmi (Bacopa monniera), Indian Journal Medical Research, 1979.

Mandukarpani, J., Use of Common I. Herb, *Indian Med. Assoc.*, 1978, 70, Pg. 177.

Appa Roa, M.V.R., et al. The Effect of Mandookarpani (Centella asiatica) on the general mental ability (medhya) of mentally retarded children. Indian Journal Medical Research, 8:9-13, 1973.

Battachary, S.K., et al. Antistress activity...from Withania somnifera, Phyto Therapy Research, (1/1), 32-7, 1987.

Nadkami, K.M., Indian Materia Medica, Pg. 1292.

Brandt, L.A., Cahners Publishing Co., The Gale Group, 2000.

Gelenberg, AJ., *Tyrosine For The Treatment of Depression.* American Journal of Psychiatry, May 1980, 137(5): 622-3.

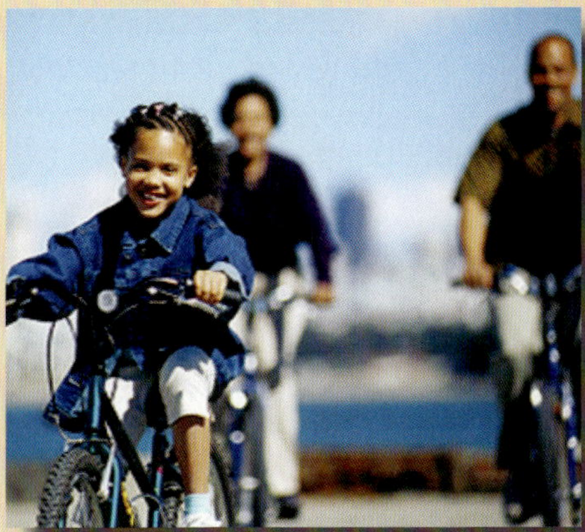
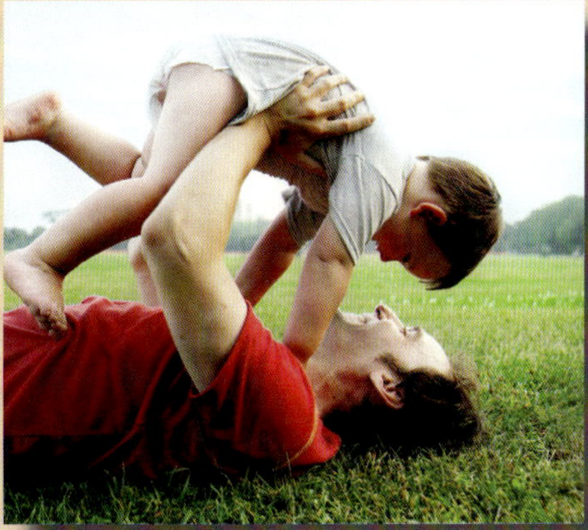
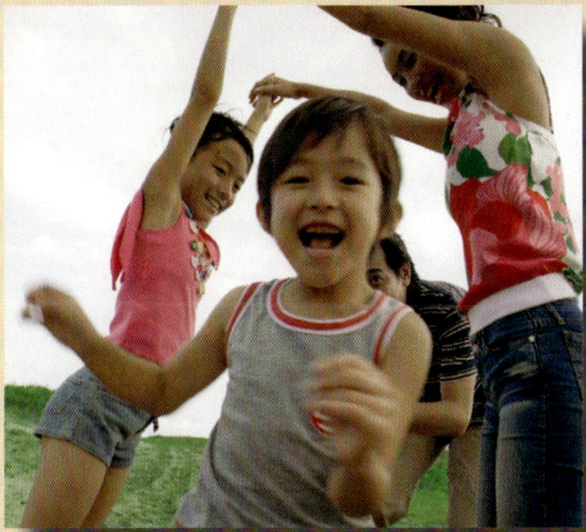
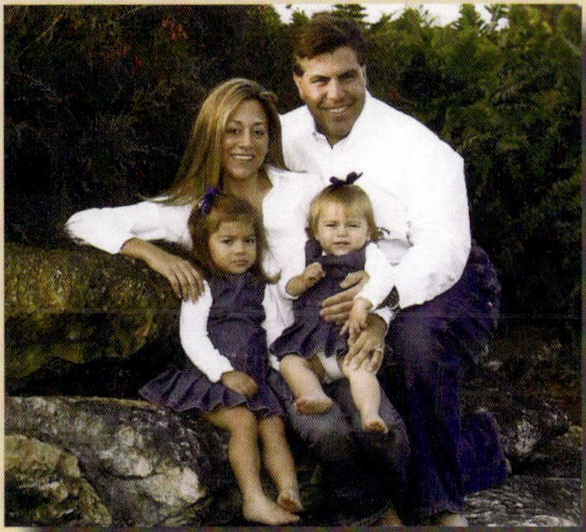

Papa Chiropractic & Physical Therapy

Providing natural solutions for more than 17 years

Dear friends,

It is our goal at Papa Chiropractic to provide you with the highest quality natural solutions and care in a professional, friendly and comfortable atmosphere. Whether you are suffering from symptoms of ADD/ADHD or other states of disease or illness, you can be confident that we will help you regain health in the least invasive and most effective ways. Our treatment programs are specifically tailored to meet your and your child's individual needs. We sincerely believe that a positive lifestyle that includes caring for your body through proper diet and supplementation, exercise, rest and enjoyment will provide you with the highest levels of health, well-being and happiness. We invite you to consider our products and services on your journey back to health.

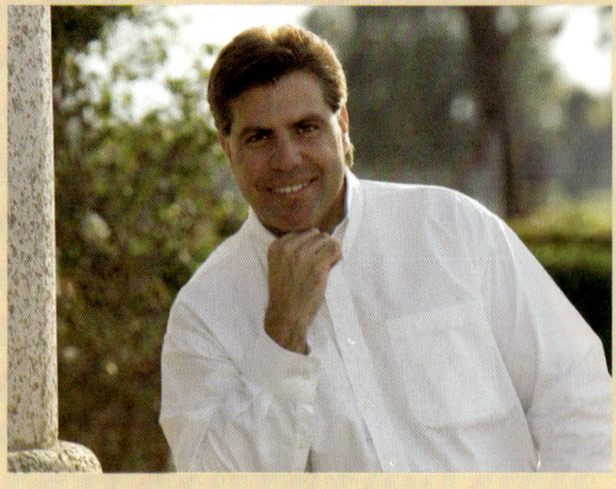

Sincerely,
Dr. Michael Papa

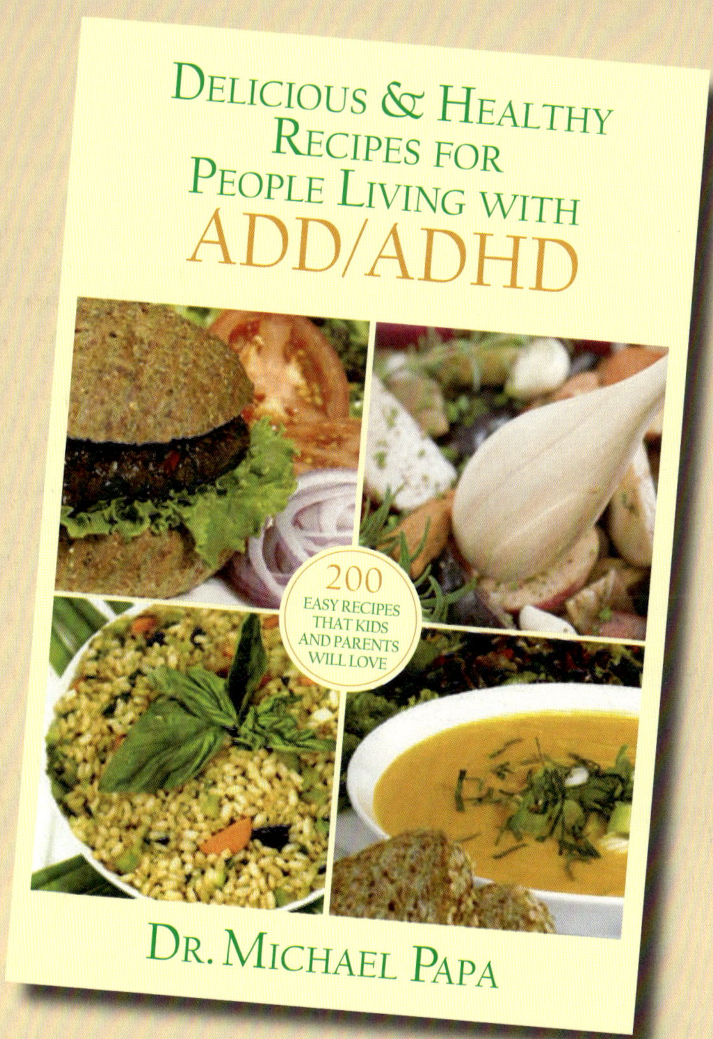

DELICIOUS & HEALTHY RECIPES FOR PEOPLE LIVING WITH
ADD/ADHD
200 EASY RECIPES THAT KIDS AND PARENTS WILL LOVE
DR. MICHAEL PAPA